The Comfort
of Home

An Illustrated Step-by-Step Guide for Caregivers

Praise for the First Edition

★★★★★ "an excellent guide on caregiving in the home. Home health professionals will find it to be a useful tool in teaching family caregivers."
—*Doody's Health Sciences Book Review Journal*

Reviewer's Choice   "Physicians, family practitioners and geriatricians, and hospital social workers should be familiar with the book and recommend it to the families of the elderly."
—*Home Care University Quality Review*

"…a masterful job of presenting the multiple aspects of caregiving in a format that is both comprehensive and reader-friendly. …important focus on physical aspects of giving care…
—*Parkinson Report*

"This book should lighten the load for anyone giving or receiving care at home."
—*InsideMS*, Theodosia Kelsy

"…almost any issue or question or need for resolution is most likely spoken of somewhere within the pages of this guide."
—*American Journal of Alzheimer's Disease*

"…particularly helpful to those who live in rural areas and do not have professionals readily accessible."
—*Western Wire*, Vicki Schmall PhD

Other Resources from CareTrust Publications:

- *La comodidad del hogar (Spanish Edition)*

- *The Comfort of Home Caregiver Assistance News* (a newsletter available in multiple languages)

- *The Comfort of Home: An Illustrated Step-by-Step Guide for Caregivers* —*Abridged Version*

- *Caregiver Training Presentation Kits*

- *Videos*

the Comfort of Home

An Illustrated Step-by-Step Guide for Caregivers

Maria M. Meyer
with Paula Derr, RN, BSN, CEN, CCRN

Foreword by Mark O. Hatfield

CareTrust Publications LLC
"Caring for you... caring for others."
Portland, Oregon

The Comfort of Home: An Illustrated Step-by-Step Guide for Caregivers

Published by: CareTrust Publications LLC
P.O. Box 10283
Portland, Oregon 97296-0283
(503) 221-1315
Fax (503) 221-7019

International Standard Book Number 0-9664767-3-5

Second Edition

Publisher's Cataloging-in-Publication
(Provided by Quality Books, Inc.)

Meyer, Maria M., 1948-
    The comfort of home : an illustrated step-by-step
guide for caregivers / Maria M. Meyer, with Paula Derr ;
foreword by Mark O. Hatfield. -- 2nd ed.
    p. cm.
    Includes bibliographical references and index.
    LCCN 98-92954
    ISBN 0-9664767-3-5

    1. Home care services--Handbooks, manuals, etc.
2. Caregivers--Handbooks, manuals, etc.   I. Derr, Paula.
II. Title.

RA645.3.M49 2002   649.8
                          QBI01-201427

Copy Editing 1st Edition: Carolyn M. Buan, Writing & Editing Services
Copy Editing 2nd Edition: Kerstin E. Meyer
Cover Art and Text Illustration: Stacey L. Tandberg
Interior Design: Frank Loose
Cover Design: Frank Loose
Page Layout: Frank Loose, Mary Sillman

Printed in the United States of America

04 10 9 8 7 6 5 4

About the Authors

Maria Meyer has been a long-time advocate of social causes, beginning with her work as co-founder of the Society for Abused Children of the Children's Home Society of Florida. She was also founding Executive Director of the Children's Foundation of Greater Miami. Maria continued her work in institutional advancement for nonprofit organizations, ranging from homeless shelters to botanic gardens. When her father-in-law suffered a stroke in 1993, Maria became aware of the need for more information about how to care for an aging parent. That led Maria to found CareTrust Publications LLC, a company dedicated to producing reader-friendly books that help ordinary people cope with their increasing responsibilities for aging family members and friends. She and her husband also founded CareTrust Services LLC, an advisory firm that helps faith-based organizations develop affordable housing and assisted living for the elderly. Maria and her husband have four children and live in Portland, Oregon.

Paula Derr has been employed by the Sisters of Providence Health System for over 25 years and is Clinical Educator for three emergency departments in the Portland metropolitan area. She is co-owner of InforMed, which publishes emergency medical services field guides for emergency medical technicians (EMTs), paramedics, firefighters, physicians, and nurses and has co-authored numerous health care articles. For Paula, home care is a family tradition of long standing. She has a special understanding of the challenges caregivers face in caring for people with Alzheimer's. For many years, Paula cared for her mother and grandmother in her home while raising two daughters and maintaining her career in nursing and health care management. Her personal and professional experience adds depth to many chapters of this book. Paula is active in several prominent professional organizations—SCCM, ENA, AACN, NFNA—and holds both local and national Board positions. Paula is a native Oregonian and lives with her husband in Portland.

Our Mission

CareTrust Publications is committed to providing high quality, user-friendly information to those who face their own aging or the responsibilities of caring for aging friends, family, or clients.

Dedication

Dedicated with loving respect to Marian, Lula, and Ciocia, caregivers of body and spirit. Their loving and selfless spirits inspire me daily. *M.M.M.*

In memory of my mother and grandmother, who lovingly allowed me to care for them in my home. *P. D.*

Dear Caregiver,

The Comfort of Home: An Illustrated Step-by-Step Guide for Caregivers is a basic but complete guide to home health care. Because health involves every aspect of living, we cover a wide range of topics, not just medical needs. You will find practical tips and illustrated solutions to help you with everyday activities, as well as with complicated and stressful situations.

The guide is divided into three parts:

Part One, Getting Ready, reviews caregiving options at your disposal; discusses the financial and legal decisions you may encounter; shows how to set up a home in a safe and comfortable way for the person whose needs are changing and abilities are declining; and, perhaps most important, shows you how to better communicate with doctors, nurses, aides, pharmacists and HMOs to get services you need.

Part Two, Day by Day, guides you through every aspect of daily care. This care may be as basic as bathing or helping someone transfer from a chair to a bed, or as adventuresome as traveling abroad with a person whose health is declining. Throughout the guide, we offer tips that will be of assistance in dealing with Alzheimer's. We also devote a chapter to understanding the stages of the disease and how to communicate with a person who has it.

Part Three, Additional Resources, provides information about the medical specialists encountered as we age; de-mystifies medical abbreviations and jargon; and includes a glossary of terms commonly used to describe and explain symptoms or conditions.

Because a picture is worth a thousand words, we frequently use illustrations throughout the guide. And we include references to helpful resources.

If "aging is not for sissies," then being a caregiver for the aging and those with special needs is not for the timid and fearful. However, knowledge will dispel your fear. With this guide in hand, you will understand what help is needed and learn where to find it or how to provide it yourself.

Warm regards,

Maria & Paula

Maria and Paula

Acknowledgments

The procedures described in this guide are based on research and consultation with nursing, medical, accounting, design, and legal experts. The authors thank the innumerable professionals and caregivers who have assisted in the development of this book. We are especially grateful to the following reviewers who made comments on sections of the manuscript during its development:

David Abrams
President
Hospice Foundation of America

Judy Alleman, RN, MN
CNS, Gerontology,
Professor, Mental Health Nursing,
Clark College

Mary J. Amdall-Thompson, RN, MS
Program Executive-Professional Services,
Oregon Board of Nursing

Julie Barsukoff Kornilkin
Caregiver

Sonya Beebe, RN
Executive Director,
Elder Abode, Lincoln City, Oregon

Brad Bowman, MD
CEO, WellMed, Inc.

Beth Boyd-Roberts, PT
Physical Therapy—In-Patient Supervisor

Karen Foley, OTR
Director, Regional Rehabilitation Services

Ruth Freeman, CNA
Caregiver

Kay B. Girsberger, RD

Deborah Hoffman

Bonnie O. Houston

Rees C. Johnson, JD

Ray Jordan, CPA

Casey C. Kellar
Author, *The Natural Beauty & Bath Book*

Esther King, RN, MN
Professor of Nursing, Clark College

Toni Lonning, MSW, LCSW
Social Worker/Care Manager

Betty McCallum, RN, BSN

Sylvia McSkimming, PhD, RN
Executive Director,
Supportive Care of the Dying:
A Coalition for Compassionate Care

James L. Meyer, AIA

Donald E. Nielsen, AIA

David E. Noble
Licensed Funeral Director and
Chairman, Oregon Donor Program

Northwest Parish Nurses Board of Directors

Cheryl Olson, RN, MBA
Director of Clinical Operations,
Home Services

Pamela Pauli, RN, MN

Lucinda J. Potter
Executive Director,
Oregon State Mortuary & Cemetery Board

David L. Sanders, AIA
President, HPD Cambridge

Annette Stixrud, RN, MS
Program Director,
Northwest Parish Nurse Ministries

James Sturgis
Executive Director, Rose Villa, Inc.

Diane Welch, RN, MN
Associate Professor of Nursing, Linfield College

We thank them for their significant contributions, without which the quality and comprehensiveness of this guide would not have been possible.

To Our Readers

We believe *The Comfort of Home: An Illustrated Step-by-Step Guide for Caregivers* reflects currently accepted practice in the areas it covers. However, the authors and publisher assume no liability with respect to the accuracy, completeness, or application of information presented here.

The Comfort of Home is not meant to replace medical care but to supplement it. You should seek professional medical advice from your health care provider. This book is only a guide; your common sense and good judgment should also be followed.

Neither the authors nor the publisher is engaged in rendering legal, accounting, or other professional advice. If legal, architectural, or other expert assistance is required, the service of a competent professional should be sought. The guide does not represent Americans with Disabilities Act compliance.

Every effort has been made at the time of publication to provide accurate names, addresses, and phone numbers in the resource sections at the ends of chapters. The resources listed are those that benefit seniors nationally, and for this reason we have not included many local groups that offer valuable assistance to the elderly and their families. Because the lists cannot include all resources helpful to seniors, failure to include an organization does not mean that it does not provide a valuable service. On the other hand, inclusion does not imply an endorsement. The authors and publisher do not warrant or guarantee any of the products described in this book and did not perform any independent analysis of the products described.

Throughout the book, we use "he" and "she" interchangeably when referring to the caregiver and the person being cared for.

ATTENTION NONPROFIT ORGANIZATIONS, CORPORATIONS, AND PROFESSIONAL ORGANIZATIONS: *The Comfort of Home* is available at special quantity discounts for bulk purchases for gifts, fundraising, or educational training purposes. Special books, book excerpts, or booklets can also be created to fit specific needs. For details, write to CareTrust Publications LLC, P.O. Box 10283, Portland, Oregon 97296-0283, or call 1-800-565-1533.

CONTENTS AT A GLANCE

Part Three *Additional Resources*

CHAPTER

Foreword

When I was invited to write a foreword to *The Comfort of Home: An Illustrated Step-by-Step Guide for Caregivers,* I had no idea that I would soon be in the role of caregiver myself. Very shortly after receiving this manuscript my wife was incapacitated at home for about a week as a result of minor surgery.

I quickly made two discoveries: First, that a major disadvantage of having a two-floor home—with kitchen on the main floor and bedroom on the second floor—is the amount of energy required of the caregiver. Second, I found that a little proverb my businesswoman wife had on her desk which said "Service is an attitude," suddenly took on a whole new meaning for me. I am fully convinced that a person must be empowered by the Divine with infinite love and compassion to carry out the many responsibilities of providing home care.

The demographics of our society are rapidly changing. Today, there are 34 million Americans over the age of 65, and the ever-increasing costs of health services make professional or institutional care impossible for most families. In fact, eighty-five percent of elder care is now provided by family members. *The Comfort of Home* will provide family caregivers with the step-by-step guides needed to successfully manage every conceivable situation relating to home care, from shampooing hair and taking care of bodily functions to managing finances and dealing with death.

I have every confidence that in writing *The Comfort of Home,* Maria Meyer and Paula Derr have compiled what will soon become the bible for the vast majority of loving, but untrained and unskilled family members providing care for their loved ones.

As a final word, I want to extend my heartfelt admiration and best wishes to each of you on the battlefront of home care. You are indeed putting love into action.

Mark O. Hatfield

Part One: Getting Ready

Part 1 ◈ Getting Ready

Is Home Care For You?

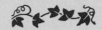

Is Home Care For You?

*T*he need to provide care for a loved one arises for many reasons. A sudden illness or hospital stay may dictate the need for help, or a person may gradually find the job of caring for a home and yard too taxing. Often, the person who needs care does not realize it and family members must step in to help with the decisions that need to be made.

One of those decisions involves who the caregiver will be and where care will be provided. The choices can be difficult unless you know the factors to consider.

Knowing What Level of Care Is Needed

Before you take on the demanding job of home care, decide what level of care you must provide. Do you need to give:

- minimum assistance?

- moderate assistance?

- maximum assistance?

- care for someone who is terminally ill?

To determine the level of care, you must understand the person's condition and needs in the areas of daily hygiene and health. Generally, these needs fall into two broad categories:

Activities of Daily Living like eating, bathing, dressing, taking medicine, and going to the toilet

Activities Important to Independence like cooking, shopping, housekeeping, getting to the doctor, paying bills, and managing money and investments

Characteristics to look for in assessing the overall level of care needed are the person's:

- ability to transfer independently from bed to wheelchair

- ability to move independently in wheelchair or walker

- ability to control bladder and bowel movements

- ability to carry out the basic activities of daily living

- ability to call for help

- degree of sight and hearing impairment

- degree of confusion

Also consider emotional conditions that might require advanced or special levels of care:

- depression

- a need for socializing or privacy

- homesickness

After giving some thought to these characteristics, try to place the person you might care for in one of these categories:

Minimum Assistance—This person is basically independent, can handle most household chores and personal care, and needs help with only one or two Activities of Daily Living.

Moderate Assistance—This person needs help with three or more Activities of Daily Living, such as bathing, cooking, or shopping.

Maximum Assistance—This person is unable to care for himself or herself, requires total assistance, and must be institutionalized if no competent and committed caregiver is available in the home. Care is often undertaken only by professionals, either in the home through home service agencies or in foster care homes, assisted living facilities, or nursing homes. At this level, serious complications are a real possibility.

Care for the Terminally Ill—This person cannot be cured and is near death. A family member can provide care at home, but it will be very difficult. If the patient has chosen hospice care, help with the physical, mental and emotional challenges is available to the patient and the family. (📖 See *Hospice Care*, Page 309.)

Deciding Whether Home Care Is Possible

When a person is suffering from chronic conditions or terminal illness, long-term skilled daily help with health and personal needs may be in order. Whatever level of care is needed, it can take place in three settings:

- the person's own home

- your home

- an institution

Home Care Considerations

Whether care will take place in your home or that of the person who needs care, the following factors must be considered:

- There is enough room for both the person and such items as a wheelchair, walker, bedside commode, and patient lift.

- All rooms are on one level.

- A doctor, nurse, or specialist is available to supervise care when needed.

- A hospital emergency unit is close by.

- The home environment is safe and supportive and stimulates independence.

- Money is available to hire additional help.

- The person in question is willing to have a caregiver in the home.

- The caregiver has few other family responsibilities.

Things That Must Be Provided

- medication
- meals
- personal care
- house cleaning

- shopping
- transportation
- companionship

- wheelchair ramps, support railings, and alterations to the bath and shower stall (☐ See *Preparing the Home, page 91.*)

Positive Effects of Home Care

- When a caregiver's spouse is supportive, the experience can strengthen the marriage.

- The relationship between the caregiver and the person in care can grow stronger.

- The savings in health care costs can be significant.

Why Home Care May Not Be Possible

- financial considerations (inadequate health insurance to cover the cost of home nursing)

- family limitations (time, money)

- the caregiver's physical and emotional strength

- the person's condition

- the home's physical layout

- the person's desire to live independent of family

Potential Hazards of Homecare

- You will lack freedom.

- Your duties may have an adverse impact on your job, career, hobbies, and personal life.

- You will have less time for family members, and your marriage may suffer.

- Children in your home will need to be quieter.

- There will be less time for religious services and volunteer work.

- Friends and family may be critical and offer unwelcome advice.

- You will often be awakened during the night.

- You may feel unable to control life's events and may suffer from depression, worry, anger, regrets, guilt, and stress.

- Instead of being grateful, the person in your care may display unpleasant changes in attitude.

- He or she may react to constant daily irritations by lashing out at you.

- You may begin to fear the time when *you* may be dependent on someone for care.

- You may feel duty-bound to spend personal funds on caregiving.

- You may become physically ill and emotionally drained.

Checklist **The Ideal Caregiver**

The ideal caregiver is—

✓ emotionally and physically capable of handling the work

✓ able to share duties and responsibilities with other willing family members

✓ able to plan solutions and solve problems instead of withdrawing under stress

✓ able to communicate in a straightforward way

✓ accustomed to giving and receiving help

✓ trained for the level of care required

✓ able to handle unpleasant tasks like changing diapers, bathing, or cleaning bed sores

✓ in good health, with energy, experience, and flexibility

✓ able to cope with anger and frustration

✓ able to afford respite (back-up) care

✓ able to communicate well with the person receiving care

✓ able to make this person feel useful and needed

✓ appreciated by other family members

✓ able to work with the future needs and preferences of the person in care

✓ aware of other care options and willing to pursue them

If you have most of these traits, you may be a good candidate to provide home care. However, consider the list of potential "hazards" on the opposite page and be honest with yourself about your ability to cope.

Outside Help

One of the biggest pitfalls in caregiving is trying to do it all yourself. But other help is available and should be called on whenever possible. That help includes:

- support groups

- day care and respite care which provide relief for the caregiver

- groups providing respite care

- pastoral counseling services

- parish nurses

- medical services provided by professionals, such as nurses and therapists

- personal care services, such as grooming or dressing, provided by home health aides

- community Visiting Nurse Association services on a fee basis

(See *Getting In-Home Help,* page 39.)

Supportive Housing and Care Options

If you believe that home care is not practical for you, many other options exist. Good programs foster independence, dignity, privacy, a maximum level of functioning, and connections with the community. However, people who have been loners all their lives may not be suited to live in groups, and those who are mentally alert may be very unhappy living with people who suffer from dementia.

Keep the above factors in mind when you check out the following alternatives:

- **Independent Living Options**—apartment buildings, condominium developments, retirement communities, and single family homes

- **Semi-independent Living Options**—places that offer the same amenities as independent living but include meal service and housekeeping as part of the monthly fee, provide help with personal care, monitor health and medications, and accommodate special diets. These options are frequently offered in Assisted Living facilities, Residential Care facilities, Foster Care Homes, and Homes for the Aged.

- **Skilled Care Facilities**—nursing homes

 States have different names for types of care facilities. Services can also be different. It is important to check with the facility and each state's licensing agency to confirm exactly which services are offered. For example, in Wyoming, Assisted Living permits unrelated people to share a room; in some other places, living spaces are not shared, except by personal choice.

A Closer Look at the Options

House Sharing—For People Who Are Fully Independent

- Two or more unrelated people live together, each with a private bedroom.

- All living areas are shared.

- Chores and expenses are shared.

Foster Care Homes—Homes in Residential Neighborhoods For People Whose Needs Vary From Assistance With Individual Services to Dependent Residents with Increased Nursing Services

- Care is given to small groups of people in the primary care-giver's home or with a live-in resident manager/caregiver.

- The home is privately operated and provides private or shared rooms with meals, housekeeping, personal care (such as bathing and dressing), medication monitoring, protective supervision, and some transportation.

- Rates vary by individual care needs and Medicaid funding is often available for reimbursements for those who qualify.

- Staff are qualified and facilities are licensed according to the level of services offered, which can include: housekeeping, laundry, personal care assistance, bathing, dressing, grooming, medication management and other medical needs, such as injections, bladder and bowel incontinency.

NOTE Some states do not license, inspect, or monitor adult foster care homes. Before selecting one, call your local Area Agency on Aging or the Department of Health for the county or state to see if any complaints have been filed against the home you are considering.

Assisted Living Facilities—For Moderate Assistance to those Who Are Frail and Usually Require Assistance with Activities of Daily Living

- Each person lives in his or her own apartment.

- An emergency staff is available 24 hours a day.

- Monthly charges are based on the level of service needed.

- Recreational activities are offered.

- Meals, housekeeping, medication management and nursing assessment are provided.

- Transportation and access to medical services can be arranged.

There is no national control or monitoring of quality for these facilities but there is state licensing and regulation. For information on a specific facility, call the ombudsman in your state or the state agency that licenses the facility.

Continuing Care Retirement Communities—For People Who Want a Range of Services from Independent Living to Nursing Home Care

- They provide a lifetime contract for care.

- They provide or offer meals and can handle special diets.

- They offer housekeeping, scheduled transportation, emergency help, personal care, and recreational and educational activities.

- Many require entrance fees that can vary significantly.

- They also have monthly fees of approximately $725 to $3,500.

- Some provide home health care and nursing home care without extra fees.

- Some charge extra for nursing unit residents.

Nursing Homes—For People Who Require Continuous and Ongoing Nursing Assistance or Monitoring

Nursing homes typically offer three levels of care:

- **Custodial**—minimal nursing, but help with hygiene, meals, dressing, etc.

- **Intermediate**—help for those who cannot live alone but do not need 24-hour nursing

- **Skilled Nursing**—intensive 24-hour nursing care

Hospice care is available in nursing homes as a covered benefit under Medicare and to Medicaid recipients in those states which offer hospice coverage under their Medicaid program.

Checklist **To Use Before Deciding on a Facility**

✔ Is a probationary period allowed to be sure a person is happy with the facility?

✔ What is the facility's refund policy regarding deposits or entrance fees if the resident dies, chooses to leave, or is asked to leave?

✔ Can a resident choose his or her own apartment? Can personal furniture be used?

✔ If the person must be away for a short time (even for a hospital stay), will the same apartment be available when he or she returns? Is there a reduced rate for extended absences?

✔ If the person marries, can the couple live in the same apartment?

✔ Can the staff handle special diets? Are meal menus posted?

✔ Is transportation provided?

✔ How many people are on staff and how much training have they had?

✔ How often and under what circumstances can staff enter the apartment?

✔ Can the resident see his or her own doctor? Who administers the medications?

✔ Is physical therapy available within the facility?

✔ Is the facility licensed to deal with a resident's declining health or must the person leave if, for example, he or she can no longer walk or becomes combative?

✔ How are decisions made when a person must be transferred to another part of the facility?

✔ Is there a 30-day notice provision for ending the agreement?

✔ Is the facility certified to accept Medicare reimbursement?

✔ Will the facility let a resident "spend down" his or her assets and go on Medicaid?

Financing Options

The choice of an appropriate housing option may depend on financing available:

- **Personal Resources**—the most common way to pay

- **Private Insurance**—helpful, but some policies limit the length of benefits, and have exclusions, waiting periods, etc.

- **Medicare**—for those 65 and older, partially pays for up to 100 days in a skilled nursing care facility after a qualifying related hospitalization of more than three consecutive days (not including the day you leave the hospital). The financing of hospice care is a separate benefit under Medicare

- **Medicaid**—partially pays for services, including Assisted Living services in some states, to the aged, blind, or disabled who have limited financial resources

(📖 See *Financial Management,* page 79.)

Points to Review Before Signing a Contract or Lease

Although it is hard to anticipate problems that may arise in a care setting, it is vital to take the following steps before signing any legal papers:

- Find out who owns the facility and review the owner's financial status.

- Ask for a copy of the contract and review it with an attorney or financial advisor.

- Do not rely on verbal promises. Make sure the contract is geared to the resident's needs.

- Read the state inspection report on the facility.

- Read all the rules and policies of the facility that are not in the contract.

- Ask to see the facility's license.

Things You Should Know About Nursing Homes

Residents' Rights in Nursing Homes

General Rights—Residents maintain all their rights guaranteed under the U.S. Constitution, including the right to vote. In addition, they can receive visitors, voice concerns, form resident councils, and enjoy informed consent, privacy, and freedom of choice.

Privacy—Roommates are the rule rather than the exception. However, residents' rooms are considered private and staff must knock before entering. Also, residents can have private visits with spouses.

Restraints—Only the resident's doctor may order a restraint as part of a care plan and must state the specific restraint's use and period of use. (Use of restraints is strongly discouraged, although not prohibited.)

Lifestyle Choices—Residents do not have as many choices as at home regarding meal times, menu choices, and times for sleep. However, facilities try to accommodate residents as much as possible.

Ability to Effect Change—Issues can be brought up to the resident council or the long-term care ombudsman.

Freedom to Leave—A person chooses to enter a facility and has the right to leave at any time regardless of what the family thinks or safety concerns. We all have a right to "folly."

NOTE The following describes general guidelines regarding a patient's rights. Contact the state agency responsible for licensure to obtain specific rules for an individual state.

The Resident's Rights When Leaving the Nursing Facility

The resident of a nursing facility must be given written notice 30 days before being moved. If there is a medical emergency, no written notice is required. Generally, a resident may be moved from a nursing facility for the following reasons:

- The person wants to be moved.

- The person must be moved for his or her own good.

- The person must be moved for the good of other residents.

- The nursing facility is not being paid (however, someone who runs out of money cannot be moved if Medicaid will pay).

- The person came into the facility for special care and that care is completed.

- The facility is being closed.

If the person does not want to leave the nursing facility, IMMEDIATELY contact the state agency responsible for licensure and/or Medicaid certification.

For Questions, Call:

- the local Area Agency on Aging

- the local Senior and Disabled Services Division of the Department of Human Resources

- the Long-Term Care Ombudsman

- the Federal Health Care Financing Administration

What Family Members and Friends Should Do

- visit whenever possible

- send cards or letters between visits

- give inexpensive gifts and treats
- if allowed by the nurse, walk around with the person when visiting so as to provide exercise
- listen to the resident's complaints
- develop a good relationship with the staff

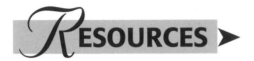

RESOURCES ▶

AARP
601 E Street, NW
Washington, DC 20049
(800) 424-3410
www.aarp.org
Website provides information on housing and other senior issues.

Assisted Living Federation of America
11200 Waples Mill Rd.
Fairfax, Virginia 22030
(703) 691-8100
Fax (703) 691-8106
www.alfa.org
Can provide a free 15-page consumer guide to assisted living and free referrals to facilities in the states of your choice.

Eldercare Locator
(800) 677-1116
www.eldercare.gov
Can direct you to the nearest Area Agency on Aging at no charge.

American Association of Homes and Services for the Aging
AAHSA Publications
901 E Street NW, Suite 500
Washington, DC 20004-2011
(202) 783-2242
(800) 508-9442
www.aahsa.org
Provides information on nonprofit organizations that offer housing and services to the elderly. Call for their free consumer information brochure. Call the 800 number to order The Consumer's Directory of Continuing Care Retirement Communities *(#CC016), a 600-page directory of 500 retirement facilities for $30.00 plus shipping.*

For a list of **Medicare Certified Nursing Homes,** call the local Office/Department on Aging.

If you don't have access to the Internet, ask your local library to help you locate a Web site.

Using the Health Care Team Effectively

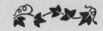

Using the Health Care Team Effectively

*W*hen you care for someone in the home, you must also manage that person's health care. This means choosing a good doctor, keeping costs down, arranging for surgery, and getting the best, least expensive medicines. It also means being familiar with the insurance rules and, most of all, being an advocate for the person in your care.

Doctors and nurses can focus on physical diagnosis and may ignore the emotional aspects of care. Sometimes they have little time to consider the spiritual aspects of healing. While you should consult with professionals about the levels of therapy and support needed for the person in your care, you do not need to accept what is recommended or ordered. Keep asking questions until you thoroughly understand the diagnosis, treatment, and prognosis.

Choosing a Doctor

Contact your local medical or dental society for the names of doctors who specialize in the field in which you seek care. Consider doctors associated with medical schools. They tend to have the most up-to-date information, especially about complicated illnesses.

- Always make sure the doctor is board certified in his or her area of specialization.

- If the person in your care is enrolled in an HMO, ask if the doctor plans to change HMOs soon.

- Be aware that you can contact more than one doctor (for a second opinion). If you are enrolled in Medicare Supplementary Medical Insurance (Part B), Medicare will pay for a second opinion in the same way it pays for other services. After Part B of the deductible has been met, Medicare pays 80 percent of the Medicare-approved amount for a second opinion and will provide the same coverage for a third opinion.

How to Share in Medical Decisions

Important medical decisions are the responsibility of the patient, doctor, and caregiver. Don't be afraid to take an active role and be an advocate for the person in your care.

Long-Range Considerations

- Find out how the person in your care feels about treatments that prolong life. Respect these views.

- Help the person receiving care set up an Advance Directive and Power of Attorney for Healthcare. (📖 See *Planning End-of-Life Health Care,* page 87.)

- Share decisions with the doctor and patient and accept responsibility for the treatment and its outcomes.

The Doctor-Patient-Caregiver Relationship

- Be aware that today doctors must see more patients per day than they once did.

- Be aware, too, that some doctors may have financial (insurance) incentives to do too much or too little for their patients—for example, to put patients in intensive care or to limit treatment. Because specialists are often the only ones who know to ask about special symptoms that pinpoint a serious or chronic condition, your doctor may refer you to a specialist.

- If your relationship with the doctor becomes unfriendly, find a new doctor.

- Respect the doctor's time (you may need to have more than one visit to cover all issues).

- Ask if the doctor accepts Medicare assignments; if not, you may have to pay the difference.

Checklist Symptoms to Report to the Doctor

*Contact the doctor **promptly** if the following changes are occurring—*

Ability to Move

✓ *falls, even if there is no pain*
✓ *leg pain when walking*
✓ *painful or limited movement (report color of skin over painful areas)*
✓ *inability to move*

Diet

✓ *extreme thirst*
✓ *lack of thirst*
✓ *unexplained weight loss*
✓ *loss of appetite*
✓ *pain before or after eating*
✓ *difficulty chewing food*
✓ *pain in the gums or teeth*
✓ *recurring gum infections*

Behavior

✓ *unusual tiredness or drowsiness*
✓ *unusual actions (aggression and anger or withdrawal)*

✓ *hallucinations*
✓ *anxiety*
✓ *increased confusion*
✓ *depression*

Bowel/Bladder

✓ *bowel movements of an odd color, texture, or amount*
✓ *a feeling of faintness during bowel movements*
✓ *vaginal discharge (report color, odor, amount)*
✓ *draining sores or pain in the penis area*
✓ *pain on urination (unusual color, amount, or odor)*
✓ *frequent urination*
✓ *frequent bladder infections*
✓ *blood in the urine*
✓ *pain in the kidney area*

The elderly are especially vulnerable to pneumonia. The flu has more severe symptoms than the common cold. It is important to call the doctor when there is a fever lasting longer than a few days, a wet cough, pain when taking deep breaths, and shortness of breath. This may be pneumonia, which can be fatal for the frail elderly.

Skin

✓ changes in the color of lips, nails, fingers, and toes
✓ unusual skin (color, temperature, texture, bruises)
✓ unusual appearance of surgery incisions
✓ sudden skin rashes (bumps, itching)
✓ pressure sores (bed sores)

Bones, Muscles, and Joints

✓ swelling in the arms and legs or around the eyes
✓ twitching or involuntary movement
✓ tingling or numbness in hands, feet, and other parts of the body
✓ warm, tender joints
✓ redness in the joints
✓ unusual position of arms, legs, fingers, or toes

Chest

✓ chest pain
✓ rapid pulse

✓ problems with breasts (report lumps, discharge, soreness, or draining)
✓ painful breathing (wheezing, shortness of breath)
✓ an unusual cough
✓ unusual sputum (report color and consistency)

Abdomen

✓ stomach pain
✓ vomiting

Head

✓ dizziness
✓ headaches
✓ ear pain, discharge, or change in hearing
✓ eye pain, discharge, redness, sensitivity to light, or blurry vision
✓ mouth sores
✓ nose pain (bleeding, unpleasant odor of discharge)

Preparing for a Visit to the Doctor

- Be prepared to briefly explain the patient's and the family's medical history.

- Take a list of questions in order of importance.

- Be prepared to ask for written information on the medical situation so you can better understand what the doctor is saying. Or bring a small tape recorder.

- You can call the hospital's library or health resource center and ask the librarian to help you look up the answers to questions the doctor does not answer.

 Be sure shots for tetanus, influenza and pneumococcal disease are up-to-date. For those over 65, influenza and pneumococcal shots are covered by Medicare.

At the Doctor's Office

- Clearly explain to your doctor what you hope and expect from treatment.

- If the doctor tells you to do something you know you can't do, such as administer a medication in the middle of the night, ask for another treatment and explain why.

- Insist on talking about the level of care that you believe is appropriate and that agrees with the patient's wishes.

- Investigate options to invasive procedures.

- Ask why tests or treatments are needed and what the risks are.

- Consider all options, including the pros and cons of "watchful waiting." (By federal law an HMO must let a doctor discuss all treatment options.)

- Trust your common sense and if you have doubts, get a second opinion.

If the Person in Your Care Is Near Death

- Because few doctors are trained to talk about death and the dying process with their patients, be prepared to begin the conversation.

- If the person in your care wants to die at home, say this clearly to the doctor.

- Be sure that any directives for health care for the person are available and prominently displayed.

(See *The Dying Process*, page 307.)

Questions to Ask Before Agreeing to Tests, Medications, and Surgery

Before you begin discussing medical treatment with the doctor, explain that you do not want any unnecessary tests or treatments. Then ask these questions:

- Why is this test needed?

- How long will it take? How soon will we see the results?

- Is it accurate?

- Is it painful?

- Are there risks associated with it? Do the benefits outweigh the risks?

- In the case of cancer, how long after treatment will unpleasant side effects occur and how long will they last?

- Are X-rays necessary?

- Will the doctor review the test report with me and explain the details?

- May I have a copy of the report to take home? (If you have concerns, ask to talk to the specialist who produced the report.)

- If a test is positive, what course of action is indicated?

- Is the condition going to worsen slowly or rapidly?

- What could happen if the test is not administered?

- How much does the test cost and is there a less expensive one?

- May I have the names of other patients you have treated for the same problem?

Questions to Ask the Doctor About Medications

Medications can be expensive, confusing to use, and have undesirable side effects. Make sure to ask questions when medicines are prescribed and prescriptions are filled.

- Give the doctor a list of all medications the person in your care is now taking including eye drops and vitamin supplements.

- Tell the doctor of any other therapies; sometimes combinations may be deadly or may keep the new therapy from working.

- Tell the doctor of any allergies or food sensitivities the person may have.

- Understand why each medication is needed and how much will it help the person's condition.

- Ask if it is possible to relieve pain almost completely, then seek the medicine that is the most effective.

- Ask how long the drug takes to work.

- Find out its side effects.

- Ask if the drug could react with other drugs and what you should do if side effects occur.

- Find out if other approaches could be used (changes in diet, exercise, stress reduction techniques, etc.)

- For a confused elderly person, ask for medicines that can be taken easily.

- If many medicines are needed, ask the doctor to prescribe them so they can be taken at the same times each day. If a drug must be taken at a difficult time (e.g., in the middle of the night), ask about another choice.

- Try to find the lowest cost alternative. Ask if a generic drug or another brand within the same drug class is available at a lower cost.

- Be sure that the generic drug will not have an adverse effect on the person's condition.

- Ask if a lower dose can be prescribed without adverse effects.

- To keep costs down, ask if a higher dose can be safely prescribed and the pill cut in half.

- Ask if you can buy just a one-week supply of a new medication until you know if the patient can tolerate any possible side effects.

PURCHASING MEDICATIONS
Purchasing medications through mail order is often the cheapest way to buy. Ask if your HMO has a mail order program.

Questions to Ask the Pharmacist

Some prescription drugs are not covered by health insurance, so it is important to shop around for the least expensive pharmacy, then stay with it. The pharmacist will come to know the patient's condition and can advise you about potential problems. Managed care plans are permitted to change medicines the doctor ordered by substituting a cheaper, but similar version. Do not try drug cost-cutting measures without first discussing the strategy with the doctor.

- When caring for a Medicare patient, ask about the government's maximum allowable charge for a particular drug.

- Ask what over-the-counter drugs the pharmacist recommends for the person's condition (it may be necessary to take more of the drug if it is over the counter).

- Ask if the HMO plan will pay for the drug the doctor ordered.

- Ask if the personal doctor will be called to approve the switch to another drug.

- Find out the generic substitute for the prescription drug.

- Ask if the generic substitute can cause adverse side effects and when the doctor should be contacted about them.

- Ask if the multiple drugs prescribed can cause potential toxic drug interactions.

- Ask if the pharmacy has a computer which will alert the pharmacist about drug-interaction side effects before the prescription is filled.

- Find out the risks of not taking the medicine.

- Find out the risks of not finishing the prescription.

- If you are caring for someone who will be taking several medications on his own, seek out a pharmacy that will do simplified packaging.

- Ask if the medicine can be put in an easy-to-open, large-size container with a label in large print.

- Ask if an overdose of the medicine is dangerous for children or a confused elderly person.

- Ask if the person can smoke or drink alcohol with the medication.

- Ask if the medicine must be taken with a meal, with water or milk, etc.

- Ask if the person can drive while on this medicine.

- When the person needs many expensive drugs, find out if you can get a discount or work out a payment plan.

MEDICAL ALERT

An elderly person who is mobile should carry a card that lists all medications he or she is currently taking.

Questions to Ask About Surgery

Surgery is a serious step to take, particularly when the patient is elderly. Ask as many questions as you need before deciding to proceed.

- Why does the person need the surgery?

- Will the surgery stop the disease or merely slow its progress?

- What are the alternatives?

- Can it be done on an outpatient basis?

- What will happen if surgery is not done?

- Where will the surgery be done? When?

- Is there a less expensive hospital?

- Will the surgeon interviewed do the surgery or will he delegate it to a junior associate? (When going into surgery, put your surgeon's name on the release form to assure that he or she will do the operation.)

- How many surgeries of this type has the doctor performed? (Generally, the more procedures of a certain type the surgeon has performed, the higher the success rate.)

- What is the doctor's success rate with this type of surgery?

- What are the anesthesiologist's qualifications?

- What can go wrong?

- How much will it cost, and is it covered by insurance or Medicare?

- What other specialists can I ask for a second opinion? (Medicaid and Medicare usually pay for second opinions. Doctors expect people to want a second opinion when surgery is needed, and they will help you get one.)

MEDICAL RECORDS

To save costs, have all medical records and tests sent to the second doctor. Also, if possible, bring the important ones with you.

Even the experts can disagree about the best treatment. The final decision is yours.

Alternative Treatments

A healthy lifestyle is now encouraged by both traditional and alternative medical providers. Medications may provide only temporary relief if ill health is caused by stress. When stress is the culprit, its source should be found. However, if you are considering alternative healthcare, ask the same questions you would ask any medical specialist. In addition:

- Be suspicious of anyone who says to stop seeing a conventional doctor or to stop taking prescribed medicine.

- Meditate or exercise regularly to help reduce the need for prescription drugs.

- Remember, most HMOs do not cover the option of consulting alternative medical practitioners.

Mental Health Treatment

Strong emotions are a normal reaction to long-term illness. Psychological counseling and support groups are an invaluable help.

- For one who is depressed and needs therapy, ask the primary care doctor for a referral to a therapist.

- Be aware that many seniors see mental health problems as embarrassing and are reluctant to seek care.

- For help determining a person's ability to make legal decisions, arrange for a geriatric psychiatrist's assessment.

(See *Depression,* page 217.)

Dental Care

As a person ages, dental care is needed more often and can become expensive. For low-cost dental programs, check with university dental schools or the local Area Agency on Aging.

- Tell the dentist all the medications the person is taking before starting dental treatment.

- If the person in your care has a chronic illness such as Parkinson's Disease, go to a dentist familiar with that disease. (Ask your local chapter or support group for a list of names.)

- Find out the minimum number of visits needed per year.

- Ask about low-cost alternatives to the recommended treatment.

- Ask if X-rays are really necessary.

- Find out the cost of dentures, but be wary of prices too good to be true. Cheap dentures may not fit correctly.

- When seeking another opinion, have all medical records and tests sent to a second dentist.

> **NOTE** If your doctor recommends a procedure and the HMO refuses to cover it, see *Appealing an HMO Decision*, page 64.

Vision Care

After age 50, regular eye exams every two years by an ophthalmologist or an optometrist are essential to detect serious eye disease. These exams can also detect other serious diseases such as diabetes. Early detection and treatment can prevent serious diseases from unnecessarily deteriorating and leading to blindness.

- Tell the doctor of any medicines the person is taking.

- Tell the doctor the family history of glaucoma.

- Get yearly eye exam for a person with diabetes.

- Contact your state's Commission for the Blind for information on self-help organizations for those with low vision.

- Insist on resources to find adaptive products (talking watches, etc.) and aids to adapt to low vision.

- Seek out radio stations that have programs of newspaper readings.

 Danger signs to watch for are changes in the color or size of an object when one eye is covered or straight poles that appear bent or wavy. See an ophthalmologist without delay.

How to Watch Out for Someone's Best Interests in the Hospital

When in the hospital, a patient is vulnerable, so be prepared to keep tabs on treatments, ask questions, and act as an advocate.

- If the Patient's Bill of Rights isn't posted in a prominent place, ask for a copy.

- Only agree to procedures that make sense to you.

- If you think a procedure is needed, ask why it is not being provided.

- Be friendly and respectful to hospital personnel; they are human and will generally respond to a positive approach with more attentive care. (However, confrontations by family members can adversely affect care because hospital staff may avoid the patient.)

- Assist with grooming and care.

- Speak up if you notice doctors or nurses doing examinations without first washing their hands.

- Check itemized bills and ask questions about unclear portions.

NOTE According to Federal law, a hospital must release patients in a *safe manner* or must keep them in the hospital. Discharge from the hospital is unwise when complications occur or when the patient has constant fever, uncontrolled infection, confusion, disorientation, inability to take food and liquids by mouth, or uncontrolled pain. In some cases, however, it may be healthier for the person to be released from the hospital because the noise and infectious diseases there may make recovery more difficult. If you plan to appeal a discharge, understand the rules of Medicare, the HMO, or your insurance plan.

When You Doubt the Time Is Right for Discharge

- State your doubts in a simple letter to the hospital's director or the health plan's medical director. (Rules vary from state to state.)

- Meet with the hospital's discharge coordinator.

- Ask if the hospital is following the usual policy for the condition.

- Explain any special circumstances that may make discharge unwise.

- Ask if the usual hospital guidelines can be modified to cover these special circumstances.

- Remember that anyone under Medicare has the right to appeal a discharge.

- Enlist your doctor's help in the appeal, but understand that the doctor may have constraints or incentives or may have a different opinion than you about the timing of the discharge.

Checklist **Coming Home from the Hospital**

✓ Assess the person's condition and needs.

✓ Understand the diagnosis and prognosis.

✓ Become part of the care team (doctor, nurse, therapists) so you can learn how to provide care.

✓ Get complete written instructions from the doctor. If there is anything you don't understand, ASK QUESTIONS.

✓ Arrange follow-up care from the doctor.

✓ Develop a Plan of Care with the doctor. (See **Setting Up the Plan of Care,** page 137.)

✓ Meet with the hospital's social worker or discharge planner to determine home care benefits.

✓ Understand in-home assistance options. (See **Getting In-Home Help,** page 39.)

✓ Arrange for in-home help.

✓ Arrange physical, occupational, and speech therapy as needed.

✓ Find out if medicine is provided by the hospital to take home. Otherwise, you will have to have prescriptions filled before you take the patient home.

✓ Prepare the home. (See **Preparing the Home,** page 91.)

✓ Buy needed supplies; rent, borrow, or buy equipment such as wheelchairs, crutches, and walkers.

✓ Take home all personal items.

✓ Check with the hospital cashier for discharge payment requirements.

✓ Arrange transportation (an ambulance or van if your car will not do).

ASK, ASK, ASK QUESTIONS UNTIL YOU ARE SATISFIED. Doctors and other health care professionals bring medical expertise, but only you can explain symptoms. Report accurately, in as few words as possible, any unusual symptoms, changes in condition, and complaints the person has.

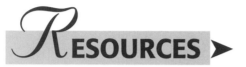ESOURCES ➤

Free or low-cost resources: local consumer health resource/information centers (check your local hospital system or phone book) and local health agencies or associations (American Heart Association, American Diabetes Association, Multiple Sclerosis Society, and others).

The Health Resource, Inc.
933 Faulkner Street
Conway, AR 72034
(501) 329-5272
Fax (501) 329-9489
(800) 949-0090
www.thehealthresource.com
Provides clients with individualized, comprehensive reports on their specific medical conditions. These reports contain treatments, both conventional and alternative, and information on current research, nutrition, self-help measures, specialists, and resource organizations. Reports on any non-cancer condition are $295, or $395 for complex issues, and contain 50 to 100 pages. Reports on any cancer condition are $395 and contain 150 to 200 pages. Shipping is additional.

Medcetera, Inc.
4515 Merrie Lane
Bellaire, TX 77401
(800) 748-6866 or (713) 664-3222
Fax (713) 666-6891
www.medcetera.com
Provides a customized research report with the latest information on any medical condition from reliable medical sources. Searches range from $89 to $135 and up.

Doctor's Guide to the Internet - Patient Edition
www.pslgroup.com/PTGUIDE.HTM
Provides information for specific diseases and gives pointers to other Internet sites of medical information.

Go Ask Alice
www.cc.columbia.edu:80/cu/healthwise/alice.html
Provides helpful information and lets you post health-related questions that will be answered for later retrieval.

University of Washington
www.washington.edu/medical
A great storehouse of general health information on all topics.

If you don't have access to the Internet, ask your local library to help you locate a Web site.

Getting In-Home Help

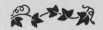

Getting In-Home Help

Getting help with caregiving in the home involves the following options:

- *Use a Home Health Care Agency (Typical Fee Range: $50–$150 per visit through a private agency)*

- *Hire someone privately (Typical Fee Range: $12 to $15 per hour—the cost of assistance is based on the category of professional)*

- *Perform all caregiving duties yourself.*

Use a Home Health Care Agency

Home Health Care Agencies are for-profit, nonprofit, or governmental. They ensure quality of care by providing personal care, skilled care, patient and caregiver instruction, and supervision. They usually provide Certified Nurse Assistants (CNAs), sometimes called Home Health Aides; Registered Nurses (RNs); Licensed Practical Nurses (LPNs); Physical Therapists; Occupational Therapists; and Speech Therapists by training. (A doctor's order is required to obtain reimbursement for skilled-care nursing in the home.) These agencies develop a plan of service to implement the Plan of Care that matches the health, social, and financial needs of the client.

Definitions for Agencies

A number of terms exist to describe agency qualifications and services. Study them carefully before you evaluate those in your area.

Accredited—Services have been reviewed by a nonprofit organization interested in quality home health care.

Bonded—The agency has paid a fixed dollar amount to be bonded; in the event of court action the bond pays the penalties. (Being bonded is not assurance of good service.)

Certified—The agency has met minimum federal standards for care and participates in the Medicare program.

Certified Health Personnel—The personnel of the agency meet the standards of a licensing agency for the state.

Insurance Claims Honored—The agency will investigate insurance benefits and will accept assignment of benefits.

Licensed—The agency has met operating requirements (in those states that regulate home health care agencies).

Licensed Health Personnel—The personnel of the agency have passed the state licensing exam for that profession.

Screened—References have been checked; a criminal check may or may not have been made.

How to Finance the Help of an Agency

Options for funding care from an agency range from Medicare to private pay or long-term care insurance.

Medicare

To be eligible for the Medicare home-health benefit, a person must be essentially homebound and need *intermittent* skilled care.

- Medicare pays the full cost of medically necessary home health visits by a Medicare-approved home health agency.

- Medicare will pay for some elderly care if the person qualifies for skilled care (expertise of a registered nurse) which is not considered maintenance.

- The patient must be as impaired as one who would otherwise be in a nursing home.

> **NOTE** States vary on eligibility requirements, so check with your area Medicare office for local rules.

Private Pay

- If a person does not qualify for public funds, he or she must pay with long-term care insurance or pay privately.

- Care management through Area Agencies on Aging may be free or offered on a sliding scale, based on a person's income.

What the Agency Will Do

- conduct an in-home visit

- investigate insurance benefits and publicly funded benefits

- ask for an assignment of benefits

- ask you to sign a "release of medical information" form

- ask you to agree to and sign a service contract

- conduct an assessment (by the director of nurses) to determine the level of care required

- discuss the various costs of suggested services

- develop a Plan of Care that shows the person's diagnosis, functional limitations, medications, specific diet, description of services provided by agency, detailed instructions for care, and list of equipment needed

- give you a written copy of the Plan of Care

- send a copy of the Plan of Care to the person's doctor

- select and send appropriate caregivers, only to the level of care needed, to the person's home

- adjust services to meet changing needs

Expect the Agency to:

- be your advocate, advisor, and service coordinator and communicate clearly with you

- provide a comprehensive assessment by professionals

- contact your doctor as part of the assessment process

- have knowledge of long-term care services and how to pay for them

- fill out the necessary paperwork for public entitlement benefits

- show no favoritism to certain service providers because of agency contracts with them

- provide confidential treatment

- provide you with written documentation of care at your request

- have a proven track record as a fiduciary agent if the agency handles a person's money

Checklist **Things to Do Before Selecting an Agency**

✓ *Interview several agencies.*

✓ *Get references and CHECK THEM.*

✓ *Make a list of services you want and ask the agency for an estimate of cost.*

✓ *Ask for an explanation of the steps in the care management process and how long each will take.*

✓ *Understand how and when you can contact the care manager.*

✓ *Find out if the agency has a system for sending out a substitute aide if the regular one doesn't show up.*

✓ *Ask if the agency will replace the aide if the person in care finds the original aide incompatible.*

✓ *Ask about the qualifications of personnel and their on-going training.*

✓ *Ask how the quality of services are monitored.*

✓ *Ask for the services the person in care needs, even if the insurance company covering the long-term care is trying to control costs.*

✓ *Be aware that if a social service agency is providing the care services, they may limit you to the particular services that they provide.*

✓ *Ask for a disclosure of referral-fee arrangements with nursing homes or other care facilities.*

✓ *Know the process for lodging complaints against the agency with the state ombudsman or long-term care office at the state level.*

✓ *Contact the local/state Division for Aging Services to check for complaints against a particular agency.*

Hire Someone Privately

Even if you decide against using an agency, a health care professional can help evaluate and prepare the home, give advice about needed supplies and where to purchase them, and set up an organized care program. However, when you hire someone privately, you must assume payroll responsibility, complete mandatory government forms (such as Social Security), determine fringe benefits, track travel expenses, and provide a detailed list of tasks to be performed.

WHEN YOU START CALLING FOR ASSISTANCE:

- Be prepared with information, such as services needed and personal information, (age of person, date of birth, social security number).
- Have your specific questions written down and ready.
- Realize that to qualify for some services there may be income, age, or geographic requirements.
- COMMUNICATE, COMMUNICATE, COMMUNICATE what you want and need!

Where to Find Help

- the Yellow Pages under Nurses, Nursing Services, Social Service Organizations, Home Health Services and Senior Services

- commercial agencies, which operate like temporary employment agencies, screen applicants, and provide you with a list of candidates

- nonprofit agencies, such as the Visiting Nurse Association, which may charge a fee on a sliding scale

- public health nursing through a county social service department (if you have no insurance or money)

- a hospital discharge planner

- hospital-based home health agencies

- the School of Nursing at a local community college

- college employment offices

- hospices (call the National Hospice Organization)

- nurses' registries

- Catholic Charities, Jewish Family Services

- the American Red Cross

- churches or synagogues

- a nearby nursing home employee who seeks part-time work

Also, consider paying an adult relative a fair hourly wage in lieu of hired services.

Categories of Health Care Professionals

Registered Nurse (RN)—has at least 2 years academic training and is licensed by the state Board of Nursing Examiners

Licensed Practical Nurse (LPN)—completes a one-year course of study and is licensed by the state Board of Licensed Vocational Nurses

Home Health Aide—has training and requirements that vary state to state; is screened on the basis of work experience

Certified Nurses Aide (CNA)—has completed 70 hours of classes and 50 hours of clinical practice in a nursing center setting; must pass a test and register with the State Board of Nursing

Someone who is in an educational or training program that leads to one of the above professions might be a candidate to help with care.

Tax Rules You Must Follow If You Hire Privately

- If you pay more than $1,100 in a calendar year, you are required to pay Medicare and Social Security tax.

- You may use Form 1040 federal income tax return to pay the Social Security, Medicare, and Federal Unemployment (FUTA) taxes. Ask Internal Revenue Service for the *Household Employer's Tax Guide.*

- For tax information, call the Social Security office; check the front of your phone book under State Government.

How to Screen a Home Care Employee

- Check licenses, training, experience, and references.

- Be sure the applicant is insured for malpractice or liability.

- Conduct a criminal background check and a driving record check (through a private investigator). Also, ask to see the applicant's insurance card.

- Find out if the applicant has a specialty (for example, terminal patients or paralysis).

- Decide whether the applicant has the personality type to meet the emotional needs of the person in your care.

- Consider the applicant's personal habits.

- Find out if he or she is a smoker or a non-smoker.

NOTE You can hire a private investigator to check public records and verify education and professional licenses, driving history, and previous employers. This service can be obtained anywhere in the country.

Ask the Applicant's References:

- How long have you known the applicant?

- Did the applicant work for you?

- Is the applicant flexible, punctual, reliable, trustworthy, patient, and courteous?

- How does the applicant handle conflicts and emergencies?

- How well does the applicant follow instructions, requests, and suggestions?

Perform All Caregiving Duties Yourself

If you decide to provide all the caregiving yourself, you can receive training at—

- social service agencies

- hospitals

- community schools

- the American Red Cross

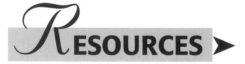

ESOURCES ▶

Family Caregiver Alliance
690 Market Street, Suite 600
San Francisco, CA 94104
(415) 434-3388
(800) 445-8106
Fax: (415) 434-3508
www.caregiver.org
E-mail: info@caregiver.org
Resource center for caregivers of brain-impaired adults. The web site provides information on services for families caring for loved ones with Alzheimer's and other brain disorders.

Eldercare Locator
(800) 677-1116
www.eldercare.gov
Provides information about local support resources providing services to the elderly.

If you don't have access to the Internet, ask your local library to help you locate a Web site.

Paying for Care

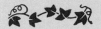

Paying for Care

*Y*ou can look to numerous sources for financial assistance. Some are public; others are private or volunteer. The most common ways to pay for home care are:

- *personal and family resources*

- *private insurance*

- *Medicare, Medicaid, Department of Veterans Affairs, and Title programs*

- *community-based services*

Assessment of Financial Resources

First, complete a Personal Financial Resources Assessment. This involves the following steps:

- Look at current assets, sources of income, and insurance entitlements.

- Prepare a budget and make projections of future income from all sources.

- Confirm the qualifications, retirement benefits, and Social Security status of the person in your care.

- Estimate the expenses of professional care and equipment (often done with the hospital discharge planner). Include any medical procedures likely to be needed.

- Check on the person's personal tax status and determine what care items and expenses are deductible.

- Determine if the person's health insurance or employer's workers' compensation policy has home health care benefits.

- Determine how much money the person will need.

 Consider making the person in your care a "dependent" and thus transferring medical expenses to a taxpayer who can take advantage of medical deductions. (📖 See *Financial Management and Tax Planning*, page 73.)

Public Pay Programs

Medicare

Medicare is a federal health insurance program providing health care benefits to all Americans 65 and older and to certain disabled Americans. Because of constant changes in Medicare policies, requirements, and forms, it is always best to get the most current information on benefits by calling the Medicare Hotline (page 68) or your hospital's social worker. No additional premium payment is required for basic Medicare coverage beyond the Social Security deduction.

General Considerations That Affect Medicare Eligibility

Whether the Person Is Homebound—Medicare will pay for certain parts of home health care only if the patient is confined to the home and requires part-time skilled (nursing) services or therapy. Medicare does not cover on-going custodial care. "Confined to home" does not mean bedridden, but it means that a person cannot leave home except for medical care and requires help to get there. (Brief absences from the home do not affect eligibility.)

What the Plan of Treatment Is—To be reimbursable, treatments, services, and supplies must be ordered by a doctor and be provided by a home health agency certified by Medicare and the State Health Department.

Whether Care Is Intermittent—Skilled services need to be irregular. Medicare is not designed to meet all the needs for chronic conditions or long-term care.

Medicare Generally Pays for the Following:

- almost all costs of skilled care, such as doctors, nurses, and specialists

- various types of therapy—occupational, physical, speech-language

- home health services

- medical supplies and equipment

- personal care by home health aides (such as bathing, dressing, meal preparation—even light housekeeping and counseling) after discharge from a hospital or nursing home

NOTE Phrases like "intermittent care," "skilled care," and "homebound" are not precisely defined. How they are interpreted has varied from region to region; the type and availability of coverage by Medicare may vary as well.

Services NOT covered by Medicare
Full-time nursing care at home, drugs, meals delivered to the home, homemaker chore services *not* related to care, and personal care services are typically not covered by Medicare. (See *Hospice Care,* page 311.)

NOTE A caregiver who has Power of Attorney for a Medicare beneficiary must submit written permission to the person's Medicare Part B carrier. Send a letter with the person's name, number, signature, and a statement that the caregiver can act on behalf of the beneficiary. The form must list start and end dates.

If there is a dispute about a reimbursement from Medicare, a review may be requested by filing a claim with the Medicare carrier.

Medicare Part B Insurance

Medicare Part B insurance costs $54.00 per month (in 2002) and supplements basic Medicare coverage. It pays for tests, doctor's office visits, lab services, and home health care. A $100 deductible applies. (These costs will increase.)

Medicare Supplemental Insurance (Medigap)

To pay for benefits not covered by Medicare, this private health insurance option is available. It pays for non-covered services only—for example, hospital deductibles, doctor co-payments, prescription drugs, and eyeglasses—but does not cover long-term care services. Coverage depends on the plan you buy.

For anyone who has Medicare HMO coverage, Medigap insurance may not be necessary because those individuals do not pay a deductible for doctor's visits—only a small co-payment.

NOTE It is illegal for an insurance company or agent to sell you a second Medigap policy unless you indicate in writing that you intend to terminate your existing Medigap policy. The federal toll-free telephone number for filing complaints is (800) 638-6833.

Medicaid

Medicaid pays for the medical care of low-income elders or those whose assets have been exhausted while paying for their own care. Eligibility must be determined, and it depends on monthly income limits and personal assets. Coverage includes both institutional care (nursing facilities, assisted living, foster care) and certain types of home care. Each state is responsible for administering its Medicaid program, so eligibility and coverage can vary from state to state. Some states have established Medicaid Waiver programs, allowing for reimbursement for home and community-based services that would otherwise only be paid if one were in a nursing home.

Common Aspects of Medicaid

- Elders must be financially and medically needy.

- For elders diagnosed as being terminally ill, benefits extend indefinitely. However, care must be provided by an agency with *hospice* certification and *Medicaid* certification.

- When a person (65 or older) signs up for hospice care, he or she gives up Medicare A and B (Waiver). Hospice care is then provided and the patient does not receive any billing. If an appendectomy or any other service not related to the terminal condition is needed, the person signs out of hospice, reinstates Medicare A and B, has the service needed and re-enrolls in hospice.

- Payments are made to providers of services on behalf of eligible elders.

- Long-term care costs are paid for those not covered by insurance and for elderly patients whose finances have been exhausted.

- Payments to foster care homes and retirement communities are not covered (except in some cases by Medicaid Waiver).

- Home health care services, medical supplies, and equipment are covered.

- Eligibility is based on a person's income and assets.

- Elders eligible for state public assistance are automatically eligible.

- Elders eligible for Supplemental Social Security (SSI) are automatically eligible.

- In many states, spousal impoverishment laws protect a portion of the estate and assets for the healthy spouse, assuming other monies are "spent down" for the care of the ill spouse. (᪲ See *General Points Regarding Asset Transfers,* page 80.)

To determine benefits, contact the local Social Security office, city or county public assistance office, or the Area Agency on Aging.

Services NOT covered by Medicaid

As a rule, Medicare, Medicaid, and private insurance do not cover many in-home services because they are not medical services. However, some community services may be called on to fill the gap on a free or subsidized basis. The following services usually are not covered but might be available locally free of charge:

- adult day care

- alcohol and drug programs

- case management

- chore services

- congregate nutrition services, such as Meals on Wheels

- consumer protection

- transportation

- emergency response systems (which provide contact by phone or electronic device to police and rescue services)

- emergency assistance for food, clothing, or shelter

- friendly visitors (volunteers who stop by to write letters or run errands)

- handicap services and equipment

- homemaker services

- legal and financial services

- mental health services

- respite care

- senior centers

- support groups (Alzheimer's, Stroke, Cancer, which will send materials if you write to them)

- telephone reassurance (volunteers who make calls to or receive calls from the elderly living alone)

NOTE The U.S. Congress and the Administration made major changes to Medicare and Medicaid, which will affect payment for long-term care. As these changes are put into effect, they are posted on the Health Care Financing Administration Web site at www.hcfa.gov or www.medicare.gov.

Department of Veterans Affairs Benefits

Veterans generally qualify for health services in the home if a disability is service related. Even if a disability is not service related, other benefits may be available based on income qualifications. Some states have special programs for veterans available only to residents of the state. Some Veterans Hospitals have programs to deliver home health care services. Contact the nearest Veterans center in your area.

Older Americans Act and Social Services Block Grant

Some agencies that provide supportive services receive funding under this program. Services available may include:

- case management and assessment

- chore services (minor household repairs, cleaning, yard work)

- companion services

- congregate meals

- home-delivered hot meals ("Meals on Wheels") once or twice a day

- homemaker services

- transportation

Private Pay Long-Term Care Insurance

Generally, private insurance programs do not cover long-term care. In many cases, home care reimbursement is severely restricted or prohibited. Policies must be examined closely. Before buying long-term care insurance, seek the best, most knowledgeable help available on the subject (for example, consult a hospital discharge planner or the Area Agency on Aging). Seek agents who represent reliable companies and have a reputation for honesty. The lack of uniformity in long-term care policies makes it hard to compare them.

- Policies vary greatly so don't assume one is like another you are familiar with.

- It's important to read the fine print.

- Such policies should not be considered an option for anyone over 79.

Checklist **Long-Term Care Insurance Policies**

✓ Look for an insurer that is top rated by Moody's Investors Service, A.M. Best Company, or Standard & Poor's Corporation.

✓ Find out how long the company has been in business and check the Better Business Bureau or the state's Insurance Division for complaints.

✓ Take someone with you when you meet the agent.

✓ Never pay cash to an agent. The payment should be made by check written to the insurance company and be sure the agent gives you a signed and dated receipt when the policy is delivered.

✓ Find premiums that do not exceed 5–6% of the covered individual's income.

✓ Ask for an "Outline of Coverage" which the law requires the insurance company to provide even if you do not want to fill out an application for insurance. Use this outline to compare policies.

✓ Understand how and when you can contact the care manager.

✓ Look for a policy that pays for care at home, in any adult foster care home, assisted living facility, and nursing home (not just one that is Medicare certified).

✓ Avoid policies that cover only skilled care. Look for policies that allow respite care and adult day care.

✓ Find out when the insurance pays for home custodial care or hospice care.

✓ Find out if previous hospitalization, a nursing home stay, or other restrictive eligibility criteria are required.

✓ Be sure that benefits will increase with inflation (5% each year).

✓ Make sure that benefits last at least three years if you don't buy lifetime benefits.

✓ Find out if some coverage is provided if the policy lapses and what conditions must be met before benefits can be started.

✓ Make sure the policy is guaranteed renewable regardless of age.

✓ Get several proposals before making a decision.

- Coverage is often limited to Medicare-certified nursing homes.

- Sometimes benefits are provided for hospice care for the terminally ill.

- Benefits are usually $50- $200 per day.

- A typical policy for a healthy 65-year-old costs about $3,000 per year.

- Long-term care insurance should be purchased before age 60, when premiums are relatively low.

- The best companies are those that offer direct cash for home care instead of reimbursement (so payment can be used for a family caregiver).

- It is important to buy what you can comfortably afford.

Long-term care insurance has two parts:

- In-home care benefits, which usually pay $100 per day for personal and domestic chores provided by a licensed home health agency.

- Nursing home benefits of approximately $200 a day.

To activate a policy, the policy holder must get confirmation from a doctor that he or she has lost the ability to do two or more of the following: bathing, eating, dressing, moving without falling, going to the toilet, and moving from a bed to a chair. The insurance company will send its representative to confirm the diagnosis. Homemaker benefits usually do not go into effect until 60 to 100 days after a hospital stay, and strict criteria must be met before in-home help is provided.

Consider Long-Term Care Insurance If:

- Personal assets exceed $100,000 for a couple or $50,000 for a single person and need to be protected.

- The assets cannot be transferred.

- There is a family history of frail-elderly.

- No one will be available to care for the person.

 Many states license individuals to offer analysis of insurance coverage for a fee. In some states if a person has a license to sell and a license to counsel, he or she can only perform one of those services for a specific client. Check your state department of insurance for information about insurance counselors.

Health Maintenance Organizations (HMOs)

Health Maintenance Organizations are prepaid health insurance plans that give complete medical coverage for a fixed premium. Knowing whether an HMO is right for the person in your care requires careful study.

Types of HMOs

There are three types of HMOs:

IPA (Individual Practice Associations) Plans—A patient chooses a doctor from a primary care physician list.

POS (Point of Service) Plans—For an extra fee a patient can visit a doctor outside of the network list.

Group Model HMOs—A patient must go to a clinic for treatment.

Remember, HMOs receive the same fees to treat a healthy person as a person with a chronic disease. For some patients with long-term or chronic illness, HMOs may not be a good choice. A patient who has a long-established relationship with a specialist who is not a member of the HMO's network list may not be able to continue to see that specialist.

> **NOTE** If a Medicare health plan is not meeting the needs of the person in your care, it is not difficult to switch to another plan or to a fee-for-service program.

How To Determine If an HMO Is Right for the Person in Your Care

- Ask if the doctor or specialist the person is now seeing is in the HMO network.

- Understand the person's medical needs—for special equipment, drugs, and help with activities. Determine if these needs are covered.

- Find out if the HMO is used to dealing with the illness the person has.

- Determine the specific services offered for this type of illness.

- Ask who decides what is medically necessary.

- Ask if there is a special Plan of Care for the illness.

- Ask if the person will get the *best* drugs for the condition or if generic substitutes will be offered.

- Ask how many people with this type of illness are under the plan in your area.

- Verify that the patient may see the specialists listed in the directory.

- Ask if the plan allows visits to specialists without a primary care doctor's referral.

- If a referral is required, find out how long it lasts and if a new referral is required for every visit.

- Ask what percentage of doctors on the list are board certified (have passed a special test given by the board of their specialty).

- Ask if the doctor has a financial incentive to do tests or to keep the patient from having tests or seeing a specialist.

- Ask if the plan covers visits to doctors outside the plan's referral list. (Out-of-network coverage may be limited to a certain dollar amount.)

- Ask how many doctors in the HMO specialize in geriatric care.

- If the person in your care must travel to a specific locale for extended stays, be sure the HMO allows visits to a different HMO there.

- Ask how the person will be charged if an emergency room visit is needed while traveling.

- Ask about the process for appealing a medical decision.

- Once you have decided on an HMO, get confirmation in writing regarding the items or services that are most important to the person in your care.

NOTE To find out how many patient complaints were registered against an HMO, call your state insurance commissioner in the phone book under State Government.

How to Appeal an HMO's Decision Regarding a Medical Procedure, Prescription, or Specialist Referral

When a treatment is denied, the goal is to reverse the denial as quickly as possible. Remember that the HMO can prolong a case in court, so the goal is to resolve the case without litigation.

- Call the HMO and ask for a copy of its formal appeals process. (Federal law requires HMOs to have such a process.)

- Make detailed notes of all conversations with the HMO; include the date and the staff person's name.

- Determine exactly why the HMO refused to cover the treatment.

- Ask the HMO clerk for an explanation; if the matter is not resolved, ask for the HMO medical director's explanation of denial of treatment.

- If you still feel the situation is not resolved, start a written appeal process.

- Ask the doctor for a written explanation why treatment is medically necessary (also ask the specialists you have visited for a letter of support.)

- Save all bills related to the problem.

- For consumer advice or support for the appeal, call the state insurance department, state health department, advocacy group for the disease, or local Area Agency on Aging.

Tip   The clerk at the other end of the line is a person too, and being courteous always gets a better response than being viewed as irrational or disrespectful.

Community-Based Services

Many services are provided free by community groups. The groups are sometimes reimbursed by state, local, and federal governments, but often it is community volunteers who provide meals and social and health care services.

These services can sometimes make it possible for a person to stay at home and maintain independence.

Typical Services

Community-based services include:

Adult Day Care Centers which provide services ranging from health assessment to social programs that cater to people with dementia or those at risk for nursing home placement

Nutrition Sites which serve meals in settings such as senior centers, housing projects, churches, synagogues, and schools, and sometimes provide transportation

Meals-on-Wheels which brings nutritious food into the home

Senior Centers which offer a place to socialize and eat (often a hot noontime meal is the only one served—and then only on weekdays)

Transportation is offered by hospitals, nursing homes, local governments, and religious, civic, or other groups. Out-of-pocket costs vary and fees are set on a sliding scale based on ability to pay.

Do These Services Meet Your Needs?

For whatever need you have, assume there may be a program servicing your area. Here are some things to think about:

- Is the person the right age and income level to be eligible for the program?

- Is it necessary for the person to belong to a certain organization (for example, Alzheimer's) before qualifying?

- Is there a limit on how many times the person can use the services of the organization?

Where to Check

- local agencies (Catholic Charities, United Way, Jewish Family and Child Services, Lutheran Family Services)

- local churches, parishes, or congregations

- the government blue book pages under "Aging" or public service listings

- city or county public assistance offices

- rural areas (call the health agency in the county seat)

- personal doctor

- family services department

- hospital discharge planner or social worker

- insurance company

- previous or current employer (may have benefits)

- public health department

- Social Security office

- state insurance commission

- state or local ombudsman

- local Area Agency on Aging (The AAA can help find available services in the community. It will know whether chore services, home-delivered meals, friendly visitors, and telephone reassurance are free of charge or are provided on a sliding scale.)

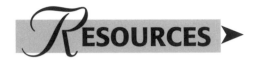ESOURCES ▶

AARP
601 E. Street, NW
Washington, D.C. 20049
(800) 424-3410
www.aarp.org
Provides information on Medicare beneficiaries.

Centers for Medicare and Medicaid Services
7500 Security Blvd.
Baltimore, MD 21244-1850
(800) MEDICARE (633-4227) Medicare Hotline
www.cms.gov or www.medicare.gov
Federal agency that administers the Medicare and Medicare pro-grams, including hospice benefits.

National Association of Professional Geriatric Care Managers
1604 N. Country Club Road
Tucson, AZ 85716
(520) 881-8008
www.caremanager.org
Provides a free list of care managers in your state by visiting the website.

The National Council on the Aging
409 Third Street, SW
Washington, D.C. 20024
(202) 479-1200
www.ncoa.org
Provides a website (www.benefitscheckup.org) for consumers that helps seniors find state and federal benefits programs.

A. B. Best
(908) 439-2200
Moody's
(212) 553-0377
Standard & Poor's
(212) 208-8000
Provide safety ratings for insurance companies you may be considering.

United Seniors Council
409 Third Street, SW
Washington, D.C. 20024
(202) 479-6973
(800) 637-2604 for orders only
www.unitedseniorshealth.org
Has information on long-term care insurance: Long-Term Care Planning: A Dollar & Sense Guide, *for $19.50, including shipping.*

For **insurance laws and regulations** call the local Area Agency on Aging or the state insurance department for counseling and information on the insurance laws and regulations governing your state.

If you don't have access to the Internet, ask your local library to help you locate a Web site.

Financial Management and Tax Planning

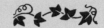

Financial Management and Tax Planning

*V*arious legal tools and tax strategies exist that can help both you and the person in your care now and in the future. Take the time to learn about them before failing health creates a crisis.

Financial management planning is an extremely important activity for each of us. However, it is not an activity to be taken without the guidance of legal and tax experts. Laws related to estate planning are complex, and detailed advice is beyond the scope of this book. Here, we merely alert you to the tools available to you. You should seek competent legal advice for your particular circumstances.

> **NOTE** Financial or estate planning is simply making sure your property—no matter how little you have—goes to whom you choose as quickly and as cheaply as possible.

Financial Management Tools

Will—a legal document that describes how money and property is to be distributed after death. A will does not cover situations where the person is disabled or incapacitated; therefore, other legal papers are needed.

Living Trust—a legal document that names someone (a trustee) to manage an individual's finances or assets. A trust includes instructions on how to manage assets and when to distribute them. It can also protect assets from probate.

Generally, the trust is activated if a person becomes incapacitated and is likely to make bad financial decisions.

Power of Attorney—a document that names someone to make decisions about money and property in the event that someone is unable to make them any longer. A person should have one power of attorney for financial management and a separate power of attorney for health care. (See *Planning End-of-Life Health Care* page 85.)

Representative Payee—someone the Social Security Administration names to manage a person's Social Security benefits. A representative payee is named when a person is unable to look after his or her own money and bill paying.

Conservatorship—a legal proceeding in which the court appoints an individual to handle another's finances when that person becomes unable to do so.

Drawing up a will, setting up a trust, providing income, and protecting assets may involve future decisions about charitable giving, insurance policies, annuities, and other instruments. This kind of planning is essential and should not be put off.

> **NOTE** Be sure to plan ahead by helping the person in your care prepare a Letter of Instructions which lists all property and debts, location of the original will and other important documents, names and addresses of professional advisors, funeral wishes, and special instructions for the division of personal property such as furniture and jewelry.

Income Tax Considerations

Under certain circumstances, caregivers can qualify for income tax benefits that offset their expenses as a caregiver. These tax "breaks" include claiming the person in care as a dependent and receiving a "dependent care credit." For the elderly or disabled person, certain tax credits also apply and some expenses are deductible.

When A Person Qualifies As A Dependent for Income Tax Purposes

Although a husband and wife are legally responsible for paying for each other's necessary health care, their adult children or other relatives are not. However, sometimes adult children and relatives provide money or resources that allow them to claim the people in their care as dependents for income tax purposes.

According to the IRS, five tests must be met for a person to qualify as a dependent for tax purposes:

1. The person does not earn more than a specified amount of gross income, adjusted each year to match the personal exemption. In 2001 the amount was $2,900. The exemption does not apply to a child under 19, or 24 if attending school.

2. The taxpayer provides more than one-half of the person's support.

3. The person has one of the following relationships with the taxpayer:

   - child

   - brother or sister

   - parent or grandparent

   - aunt, uncle, niece, or nephew

   - son-in-law, daughter-in-law, father-in-law, mother-in-law, brother-in-law, sister-in-law

   - a descendant of a child (grandchild, great grandchild)

   - step-child, step-sibling, or step-parent

OR

- any person who lives in the taxpayer's home during the entire tax year and is a member of the taxpayer's household.

4. The person did not file a joint return with a spouse.

5. The person is a citizen, national, or resident of the United States, or a resident of Canada or Mexico at some time during the calendar year, or an alien child adopted by and living with a U.S. citizen.

Tax Credit for the Elderly or Disabled

A tax credit may be available to persons who are 65 or over or who are permanently or totally disabled. Special rules and procedures apply for calculating the amount of the credit. See IRS Schedule R (Form 1040) or Schedule 3 (Form 1040A).

Some life insurance policies provide tax-free benefits (accelerated death benefits). Check with the life insurance company for details.

What Can Be Deducted for Income Tax Purposes

If a person can be claimed as a dependent and the caregiver itemizes, the caregiver may include medical expenses paid for the dependent on the caregiver's schedule of itemized deductions. If all medical expenses of the caregiver exceed 7.5% of the adjusted gross income, a deduction will be allowed.

Other deductible medical expenses are:

- improvements and additions to the home that are made for medical care purposes. (These are deductible only to the extent that they exceed the value added to the house. The entire cost of an improvement that does not increase the value of the property is deductible.)

- expenses of a dog for the blind or deaf

- lodging while away from home for (and essential to) medical care. (The deductible expenses cannot exceed $50 per individual per night. Meals are not deductible.)

- medical insurance (including premiums paid under the Social Security Act relating to supplementary medical insurance for the aged.)

- long-term care insurance premiums (subject to limitations)

- nursing homes (The entire cost of maintenance, including meals and lodging, is deductible if the primary reason one is there is because of a physical condition that requires the medical care provided.)

- Transportation costs for medical care, whether around the corner or across the country. (To determine the amounts, use the actual expenses for air fare, gas, etc., or in the case of your own vehicle, you may use the standard mileage rate of ten cents per mile.)

See your tax preparer for rules on your particular situation.

STORING DOCUMENTS

Store—Death certificates, military records, six years of tax returns, documents regarding pensions

Keep in the safe-deposit box—Original will, deeds, passport, stock and bond certificates, birth and marriage certificates, insurance policies

Keep at home— a copy of the will, leaving the original in the safe deposit box

Throw out—expired insurance policies, non-tax related checks more than one year old

Funeral Expenses

Generally, funeral expenses are not deducted for income tax purposes but are deducted if an estate tax return is filed.

Year-End Tax Strategies for Family Caregivers

As early as possible, consider the following money-saving strategies and, if appropriate, discuss them with the person in your care.

- Pay or charge medical expenses in the year when the deduction will result in a benefit. Consider bunching medical deductions in one year. (For example, buy January's prescription drugs in December.)

- See if you qualify as head of household on the tax form.

- Consider transferring, to a beneficiary, title to the property that belongs to the person in your care. This makes sense when the beneficiary could claim expenses, such as real estate taxes, that the person in care couldn't claim because of a low income level.

- Determine who should pay medical bills by figuring out who will receive a tax deduction from the payment.

- Before selling assets to care for a parent, consider the tax that will have to be paid on the sale. Decide which assets have a high basis or a low basis (original purchase price), because capital gains should be kept low. Consider gifting first to the parent and having the parent sell at a lower tax rate.

- Consider giving property of the person in your care to a charity—and doing so in a way that provides a higher income each year than he or she would receive from interest on an investment.

> **TRACKING TAX-RELATED EXPENSES**
>
> - Use a file box for storage.
>
> - Set up a separate accordian-style folder with monthly tabs for each doctor, lab, medicine, and hospital.
>
> - Keep all bills in the designated folder filed by month.
>
> - Note on the bill the check number, date, and amount paid for each bill. (Pay medical bills by check and not by credit card to keep a better record.)
>
> - Keep a daily diary of cash expense, mileage, and other travel costs for medical appointments. Hand Held Devices such as a Palm Pilot are excellent for keeping this information and also are handy for keeping a list of issues to discuss with the caregivers. You can print these lists out before visiting the caregiver to help stay on track.

Social Security Benefits

As a result of 1996 federal tax laws, people between the ages of 65 and 69 can begin to earn increasing amounts of money each year without losing their Social Security benefits. The top amount is $30,000 in 2002.

Above those limits, people will lose $1 in benefits for every $3 in wages or self-employment income earned. Call your local Social Security office to find out the current amount you can earn without losing benefits.

Understanding Social Security

- Retirement checks are loosely tied to how much was paid into the system.

- Social Security redistributes the wealth to protect people who become disabled, and it protects spouses and children of a recipient who dies. The death benefit is $225. (See *Funeral Arrangements*, page 325.)

- Social Security typically pays $858 a month for a person who retires at 65.

- Social Security, personal savings, and employers' pensions together provide financial support in old age.

> **NOTE** Name the personal representative as co-renter of the safe deposit box if the person in your care does not have a spouse or close relative to make it easier to access the safe deposit box after death.

Medicaid Guidelines

The cost of nursing home care is high and can easily wipe out a couple's savings even if only one person is in the nursing home.

Currently, Medicaid rules allow a person:

- to keep a home if he or she plans to return there or if it is occupied by a spouse or a disabled or minor child

- to have a maximum individual income (which varies state to state), including pension payments and Social Security

- to have a prepaid funeral fund of $1,500

- to have a maximum bank account of $2,000

General Points Regarding Asset Transfers

- Transfers must happen at least 36 months before applying to a nursing facility. (Transfers within 36 months will delay eligibility for Medicaid, and certain transfers from trusts can delay eligibility for up to 60 months.)

- A home can be transferred within 36 months if it is transferred to a spouse, a minor, or a disabled child.

- Transfers of assets to a child may be risky if the child will not be able or willing to help the parent if extra money is needed.

- A trust may be a better option because the money is still available for the parents' needs.

- If a person sets up a special needs trust for himself, the assets must still be spent down to qualify for Medicaid payment for nursing home care.

- Among the penalties for people who transfer assets for less than fair market value to qualify for Medicaid is a $10,000 fine and up to a year in prison.

- The healthy spouse of a person who applies for Medicaid may retain some income and resources. Each case is assessed after the applicant becomes eligible for Medicaid.

- The maximum individual income a person can have and still qualify for Medicaid varies from state to state. The rules can be complicated. In order to consider all the aspects fully, seek the advice of a competent attorney.

Abuse from Financial Advisors

Aggressive marketing to the elderly is becoming increasingly common. Although seminars for estate planning can provide useful information, they are often selling something and therefore do not offer an unbiased assessment of what a person may need. Help the person in your care avoid financial planners who may also be stock brokers or insurance agents. Before selecting a financial planner, one should always:

- Check with the local Area Agency on Aging and other agencies that work with the elderly for a list of referrals.

- Interview the financial planner and check his or her credentials (law, accounting degrees, continuing education in financial planning for the retired).

- Find out what the financial advisor will gain from your business in fee and commission income.

- Take this information into account before acting on any recommendation to buy.

- Ask for the fees in writing.

- Ask if local law requires that any comparisons of plans be provided.

- Ask if the advisor is registered with the Securities and Exchange Commission. (See *Consumer Fraud*, page 221.)

Neither the authors nor the publisher is engaged in rendering legal or tax advisory service. The information in this Guide is intended to give information of a general character only. For a correct interpretation of the way these matters affect you, please consult a CPA, attorney, or other professional advisor.

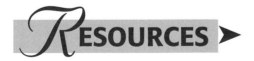

RESOURCES ▶

AARP
(800) 424-3410
www.aarp.org
Provides information on elder care issues.

Children of Aging Parents

1609 Woodbourne Road, Suite 302A
Levittown, PA 19057
(215) 945-6900
Fax (215) 945-8720
(800) 227-7294
www.CAPS4caregivers.org
A national nonprofit resource and referral organization which provides caregivers with information and referrals, a network of support groups, and publications and programs that promote public awareness of the needs of caregivers.

Social Security Administration

(800) 772-1213
Provides a personalized report on a person's Social Security record. (See *Funeral Arrangements*, page 325 for details.)

Financial Planning Association

3801 E. Florida Avenue
Suite 708
Denver, CO 80210
Fax: (404) 845-3660
(800) 322-4237
www.fpanet.org
Provides a list of certified financial planners in your region, biographies of each, and a helpful free pamphlet, Selecting a Qualified Financial Planning Professional, *which lists questions you should ask a financial planner before hiring him or her.*

Certified Financial Planners Board of Standards

(303) 830-7500
(800) 487-1497
www.cfp-board.org
To check the status of a financial planner. Organization will provide information on whether a planner is certified, how long he/she has been certified, and if any disciplinary action was ever taken .

AARP Tax-Aide

www.aarp.org/taxaide/home.htm *(for a listing of site locations)*
(888) 227-7669
Call 24 hours a day, 7 days a week to find a site near you. Provides free help on federal, state and local tax returns to middle- and low-income persons aged 60 years and older; also provides online counselors at the Web site. This program also accepts volunteers.

IRS Web Site

(800) 829-3676 for publications
(800) 829-1040 for answers to tax questions
www.irs.gov
The website provides tax forms. Form 559 is for survivors, and Form 524 is for the elderly or disabled.

Older Women's League

666 11th Street, NW
Suite 700
Washington, D.C. 20001
(800) 825-3695
(202) 783-6686
www.owl-national.org

If you don't have home access to the Internet, ask your local library to help you locate any Web site.

Planning End-of-Life Health Care

Planning End-of-Life Health Care

*I*n addition to deciding how to pay for long-term care and estate planning (topics covered in the last two chapters), it is important to decide how future health care decisions will be made **before** any condition reaches the crisis stage.

These decisions should be recorded in legal documents for two reasons:

- to make sure that a patient's wishes are honored

- to protect the family from having to make life and death decisions without sufficient information about those wishes

The capacity to plan for health care decisions depends on one's ability to:

- understand the nature of treatment choices that are available

- appreciate the implications of the various alternatives

- make and communicate a thoughtful choice

- express values and goals

Once these matters are understood, various legal documents can be drawn up to help insure that the person's wishes will be carried out.

The following information is not intended as legal advice. Rather, we have presented a general summary of the rights of competent adults to make, or arrange for others to make, their health care decisions. Our summary does not contain all the technical details of laws in each state. Check the requirements of your individual state statute.

Directives for Health Care

Two types of legal documents exist to indicate a person's instructions for end-of-life health care. One type outlines *the kind* of medical attention desired, while the other *names another person* who can make sure these wishes are carried out. (These legal documents have a variety of names, so the ones we employ below may not match those used in your state.)

Living Will

A living will is a document that details a person's wishes about medical care at the end of his or her life in the event the person becomes incapacitated and is unable to provide instructions. The living will usually directs that the process of dying should not be prolonged and that comfort should be maintained while illness takes a natural course. When developing a living will, it is important to consider a person's attitude towards lifetime nursing home care. (See *Special Challenges*, page 230, for having one's wishes honored while traveling.)

Health Care Proxy (Health Care Power of Attorney or Advance Directive)

This document allows a person to name someone as a personal representative (the health care proxy or representative) and gives that person the authority to carry out the dying person's wishes, as outlined in the living will.

Do Not Resuscitate Order (DNR)

A third document instructs medical personnel not to use CPR (cardio-pulmonary resuscitation) if the person's heart stops beating.

Values History

A fourth document explains a person's views on life and death and his or her priorities in ways that can help the health care proxy interpret those wishes. It is a helpful document to have because every possible medical situation cannot be foreseen.

Advantages of Preparing These Directives

- They can be flexible and tailored to an individual's wishes.

- They apply to all health care situations.

- They may be given to anyone—a friend, relative, or spiritual advisor—to hold until needed.

- They are honored in the state where they were written and in most other states (check the state in question).

- They are not limited to life prolonging issues but can also, for example, cover dentistry and invasive surgery.

- They can be created by filling in a standard form.

- Advance Health Care Directive forms vary from state to state and are available from most hospitals and nursing homes.

- They can be revoked at any time as long as the person is mentally competent.

Checklist **Dos and Don'ts in Planning Health Care**

✓ *Do execute a new power or directive every few years to show the intention still holds.*

✓ *Do use the approved form for your state.*

✓ *Do have the document drawn up by lawyer so it conforms with state rules.*

✓ *Do give a copy to the doctor, hospital, and any person holding power of attorney.*

✓ *Do ask the doctor and lawyer of the person in your care to review the document while that person is competent. Make sure they accept its intent.*

✓ *Do keep a card with health care information in your wallet or that of the person in your care.*

✓ *Don't name the doctor as having power of attorney.*

✓ *Do carry a copy of the document with you when you travel.* (📖 *See* **Travel**, *page 230.)*

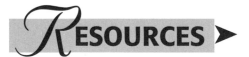

ℛESOURCES ➤

The Living Bank
(800) 528-2971
www.livingbank.org
Registry and referral service for people wishing to donate organs, tissues or whole bodies for transplantation or research.

PBS "Before I Die: Medical Care and Personal Choices"
www.pbs.org/bid
OR
www.wnet.org/bid

The Robert Wood Johnson Foundation
www.rwjf.org
OR
www.lastacts.org

Partnership for Caring: America's Voices for the Dying
1035 30th Street, NW
Washington, DC 20007
(202) 338-9790
(800) 989-9455
www.partnershipforcaring.org
For a small fee distributes state-specific forms and explanatory guides for creating a living will.

AARP
(800) 424-3410
http://www.aarp.org
Can direct you to a hotline available in some states for brief legal advice by telephone to those 60 and older.

Administration on Aging
www.aoa.gov/legal/hotline.html
Website lists legal hotlines for the states that have them for those 60 and older.

National Academy of Elder Law Attorneys
1604 N. Country Club Road
Tucson, AZ 85716
(520) 881-4005
www.naela.org
For a $25 fee you can obtain a list of member lawyers in your area and the free brochure, Questions and Answers When Looking for An Elder Law Attorney.

The Equal Justice Network
www.equaljustice.org/hotline
A website sponsored by programs in the field offering legal advice over the telephone.

Preparing the Home

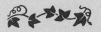

Preparing the Home

A dapting the home for a person who is partially or fully disabled can be a demanding or a relatively simple process. In general, the more adaptations that can be made early on—with a view toward future needs—the easier life will be for everyone concerned. Few caregivers can afford to substantially remodel a home. Nonetheless, we believe it is important for our readers to be aware of the "ideal" as they plan the alterations that are realistic in their situations.

Here we present suggestions—from architects who specialize in elder care housing, occupational therapists, and others—for achieving the best home care conditions.

Safety, Safety, Safety

"Unintentional injury, which often results from a fall, ranks as the sixth leading cause of death among people over 65 years of age." (*The New England Journal of Medicine, September 29, 1994*)

The first priority in preparing any home is safety. Accidents do happen but, with a little planning, are preventable. Take an objective look at the home where you will provide care. Ask a relative or friend to survey it with you to help see safety hazards you may have overlooked.

> **NOTE** Leave a blanket, pillow, and phone on the floor so, in case of a fall, the person in your care can stay warm and call for help.

As you plan for safety in the home, consider both current demands and future needs. For example, furniture that works well for a 65-year-old may need to be modified or replaced later when the person loses the strength to get up from low seats. Your first priority is to make the home as safe as possible.

As you make changes to the home, don't forget your own comfort and convenience. Making life easier for yourself means you will have more time to provide care or to rest. In the long run, this will improve the overall environment for care.

The Home Environment

The ideal home for the care of the elderly or disabled is on one level (ground floor). Multiple floors are tolerable only if they are serviced by an elevator or another approved lift device. The ideal care home is laid out in such a way that allows the caregiver and the person in care to see each other from various rooms.

Safety

For the safest home, implement as many of these steps as possible:

- Remove all unnecessary furniture.

- Arrange the remaining furniture, providing ample space for a walker or wheelchair, thus avoiding the need for an elderly or disabled person to move around coffee tables and other barriers. Move low tables that are in the walk path.

- Do not rearrange furniture after the person in your care has grown accustomed to its placement.

- Adjust furniture so it will not move if leaned on.

- Ensure that a favorite chair has arm rests that are long enough to help the person get up and down.

- Modify or cushion sharp corners on furniture, cabinets, and vanities.

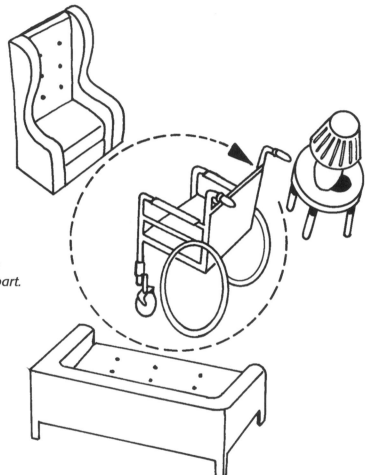

▶ *To accommodate a wheelchair, arrange furniture 5 ½ feet apart.*

- Make chair seats 20" high. (Wood blocks or a wooden platform can be placed under large, heavy furniture to raise it to this level.)

- Have a carpenter install railings in places where a person might need extra support. (A carpenter can insure that railings can bear a person's full weight and will not give way.)

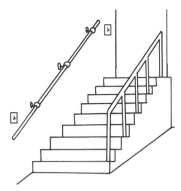

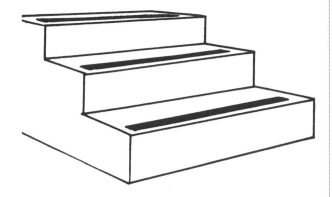

▶ *Place non-skid tape on the edges of steps.*

▲ *Always provide railings along stairs. When possible, extend the hand rail past the bottom and top step.*

- Place masking or colored opaque tape on glass doors and picture windows.

- Use automatic night lights in the rooms used by the person in your care.

- Clear fire escape routes.

- Provide smoke alarms on every floor and outside every bedroom.

- Place a fire extinguisher in the kitchen.

- Consider the need for monitors and intercoms.

- Place non-skid tape on the edges of stairs (consider painting the edge of the first and last step a different color from the floor).

> **NOTE** For a safer home environment for the person with a respiratory condition such as asthma, emphysema, or chronic bronchitis, avoid—
>
> - rugs
> - belt-type humidifiers
> - overstuffed furniture
> - books and book shelves
> - pets and stuffed toys
> - pleated lampshades
> - dirty heat ducts and air filters
> - tobacco smoke
> - wool blankets and clothing

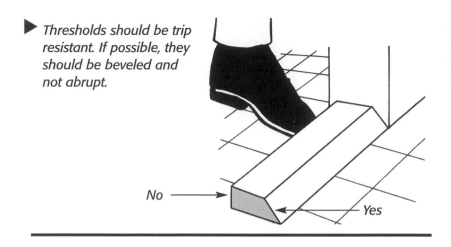

▶ *Thresholds should be trip resistant. If possible, they should be beveled and not abrupt.*

No ——→

Yes

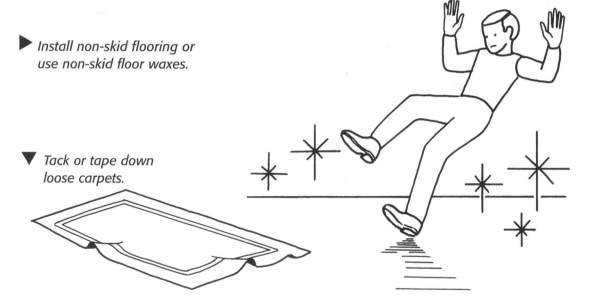

▶ *Install non-skid flooring or use non-skid floor waxes.*

▼ *Tack or tape down loose carpets.*

- Thin pile carpet is easier to walk on than thick pile. Avoid "busy" patterns.

- Be sure stairs have even surfaces with no metal strips or rubber mats to cause tripping.

- Remove all hazards that might lead to tripping.

- Secure electrical and telephone cords to walls.

- Adjust or remove rapidly closing doors.

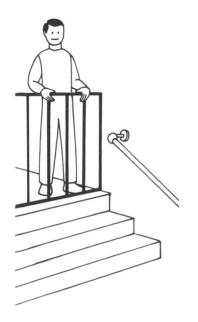

▲ *A safety gate at the top of stairs can prevent falls.*

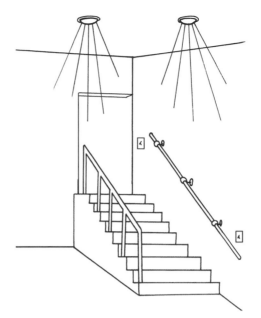

▲ *Be sure steps are well lighted with light switches at both the top and bottom of the stairs.*

- Place protective screens on fireplaces.
- Cover exposed hot water pipes.
- Provide adequate non-glare light—indirect is best.
- Place light switches next to room entrances so the lights can be turned on before entering a room. Consider "clap-on" lamps beside the bed.
- Use 100–200 watt light bulbs for close-up activities (but make sure lamps can handle the extra wattage).

NOTE An 85-year-old needs about three times the amount of light a 15-year-old needs to see the same thing. Contrasting colors are a big part of seeing well. As much as possible, have furniture, toilet seats, counters, etc. a different color than the floor.

- Plan for extra outdoor lighting for good nighttime visibility, especially on stairs and walkways.

- If possible, install a carbon monoxide detector that sounds an alarm when dangerous levels of CO are reached. Call the **American Lung Association**, (800) LUNG USA, for details.

- Develop an emergency evacuation plan in case of fire.

> **NOTE** If the person in your care is on life support equipment, install a back-up electrical power system and have a plan of action for a power outage.

Comfort and Convenience

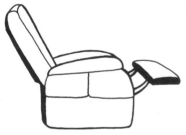

▲ *Consider a power-assisted recliner that allows the power-assist feature to be turned off.*

- For frail or wheelchair-bound persons, install automatic door operators (system of pulleys and weights or electro-mechanical openers that plug into outlets).

- For a person with a wheelchair or a walker, allow at least 18–24" clearance from the door on landings.

- Plan to leave ample space (a minimum of 32" clear) for moving a hospital bed and wheelchair through doorways.

▶ *Install entry ramps. Rails can be added for additional safety.*

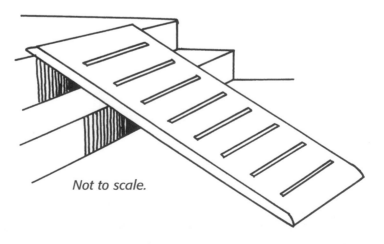

Not to scale.

> **NOTE** If you are remodeling a two-story house, have the contractor frame in the shell of the elevator and then add the elevator unit later when needed. Use the space as a closet now.

- To widen doorways, remove the molding and change regular door hinges to offset hinges. Whenever possible, remove doors.

- Install lever handles on all doors.

- If a disabled person must be moved from one story to another, install a stair elevator.

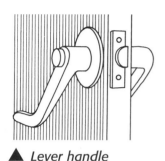

▲ *Lever handle*

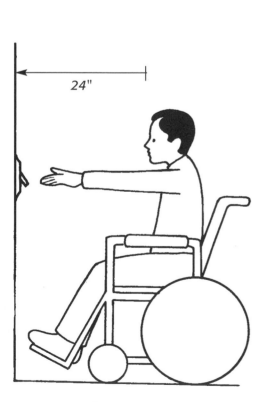

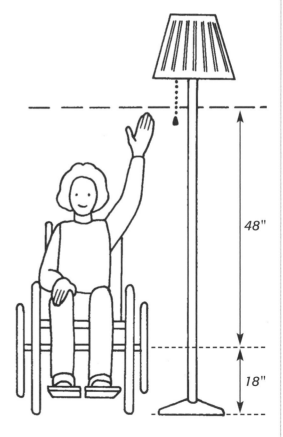

▲ *A person can reach forward about 24" from a seated position. Between 18" and 48" from the floor is the ideal position for light switches, telephones, and mail boxes.*

The Bathroom

Many accidents happen in bathrooms, so check the safety of the bathroom that you will use for home care.

Safety

▶ *Install grab bars beside the toilet, along the edge of the sink, and in the tub and shower according to the needs of each individual.*

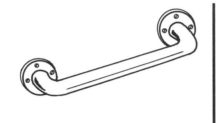

▶ *Five inch door pulls or utility handles can be installed on door frames and window sills.*

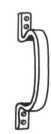

- Cover all sharp edges with rubber cushioning.

- Install lights in medicine cabinets so mistakes are not made when taking medicine.

- Remove locks on bathroom doors.

- Use non-skid safety strips or a non-slip bath mat in the tub or shower.

- Consider installing a grab rail on the edge of the vanity. (Do not use a towel bar.)

- Remove glass shower doors or replace them with unbreakable plastic.

- Use only electrical appliances with a Ground Fault Interrupted (GFI) feature.

- Install GFI electrical outlets.

- Set the hot water thermostat below 120° F.

- Use faucets that mix hot and cold water, or paint hot water knobs/faucets red.

- Insulate hot water pipes to prevent burns.

- Install toilet guard rails or provide a portable toilet seat with built-in rails. (📖 See *Equipment and Supplies*, page 122.)

Comfort and Convenience

- If possible, have the bathroom in a straight path from the bedroom of the person in your care.

- Install a ceiling heat lamp.

- Place a telephone near the toilet.

- Provide soap on a rope or put a bar of soap in the toe of a nylon stocking and tie it to the grab bar.

- Place toilet paper within easy reach.

- Try to provide enough space for two people at the bathroom sink.

- If possible, have the sink 32" from the floor.

- On faucets, use levers instead of handles.

- Provide an elevated toilet seat.

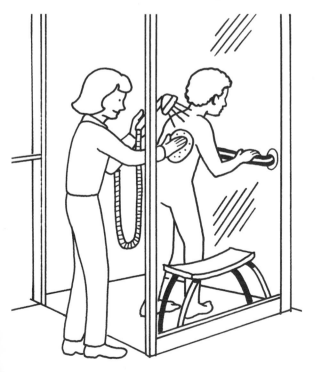

◀ *If possible, have a shower stall that is large enough for two people. Use a hand-held shower head with a very long hose and an adjustable jet stream. Provide a tub seat or bench in the shower stall.*

The Kitchen

Many of the following suggestions are made to fit the needs of handicapped or elderly people who are able to help in the kitchen.

Safety

- Use an electric tea kettle.

- Set the water heater temperature at 120° F.

- Use a single lever faucet that can balance water temperature.

- Provide an area away from the knife drawer and the stove where the person in your care can help prepare food.

- Use a microwave oven whenever possible (but not if a person with a pacemaker is present).

- Ask the gas company to modify your stove to provide a gas odor strong enough to alert you if the pilot light goes out.

- If possible, have the range controls on the front of the stove.

- Provide a step stool, never a chair, to reach high shelves.

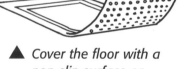

▲ *Cover the floor with a non-slip surface or use a non-skid mat near the sink, where it may be wet.*

Comfort and Convenience

- Use adjustable-height chairs with locking casters.

- Install Lazy Susans® (swivel plate) in corner cabinets.

- Rearrange cabinets to reduce bending and reaching.

- Install a storage wall rather than upper cabinets.

- For easy access, replace drawer knobs with handles.

- To reduce back strain from reaching dishes, place a wire rack on the counter.

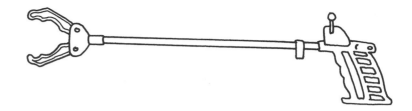

▶ *Use reachers—devices for reaching objects in high or low places without stretching, bending, or standing on a stool.*

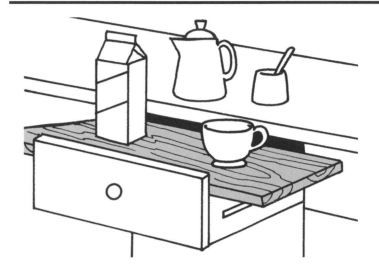

▶ *A cutting board placed over a drawer provides an easy-to-reach surface for a person in a wheelchair.*

- Adapt one counter for wheelchair access as pictured above.

- Remove doors under the sink to accommodate a wheelchair; also insulate exposed pipes.

- Create different counter heights by installing folding or pull-out surfaces.

- When bending is difficult, consider a wall oven.

- Use drawer suspension systems for heavy drawers.

- Install pull-out shelves in cabinets.

- If possible, use a refrigerator with the freezer on the bottom.

- Prop the front of the refrigerator so the door closes automatically. (If necessary, reverse the way the door swings.)

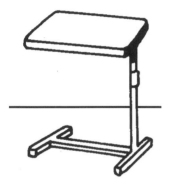

> **NOTE** To reduce the chance of falls and to avoid reaching and bending, place frequently used items at a level between the shoulders and knees.

The Bedroom

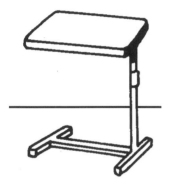

▲ *Provide an adjustable over-the-bed table of the type used to serve meals in hospital rooms.*

Ideally provide 3 bedrooms, one for the person in care, one for yourself, and one for the home health aide. Also—

- Install a monitor to listen to activity in the room of the person in your care. (Some are inexpensive and portable.)

- Make the bedroom bright and cheerful.

- Make sure adequate heat (65° F at night) and fresh air are available.

- Provide a firm mattress.

- Provide TV and radio.

- Consider a fish aquarium for distraction and relaxation.

- Use disposable pads to protect furniture.

- Install room-darkening blinds or shades.

- Place closet rods 48" from the floor.

- Provide a chair for dressing.

- Keep a flashlight at the bedside table.

- Provide a bedside commode with a 4" foam pad on the seat for comfort.

- Hang a bulletin board with pictures of family and friends where it can be easily seen.

- Provide a sturdy chair or table next to the bed for help getting in and out of bed.

- Make the bed 22" high and stabilize it against a wall or use lockable wheels to allow the person who uses it to get up and down safely.

- Use blocks to raise a bed's height, but be sure to stabilize them carefully.

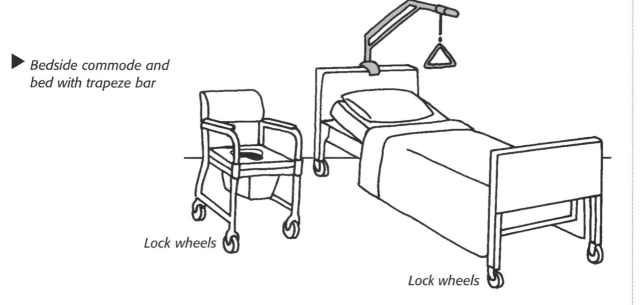

▶ *Bedside commode and bed with trapeze bar*

Lock wheels

Lock wheels

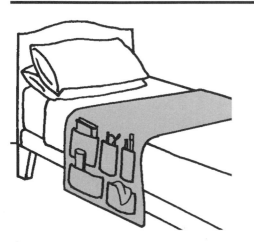

▲ *Make a bed organizer to hold facial tissues, lotion, and other items needed at the bedside by attaching pockets to a large piece of fabric spread across the bed.*

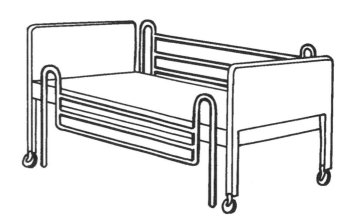

▲ *When all the care is at the bedside, consider a hospital bed—helpful for both you and the person in your care.*

The Telephone

Contact your local phone company's special needs department or visit a store that sells phones and related accessories to inquire about:

- increasing the number size on your phone dial for improved visibility and ease of use

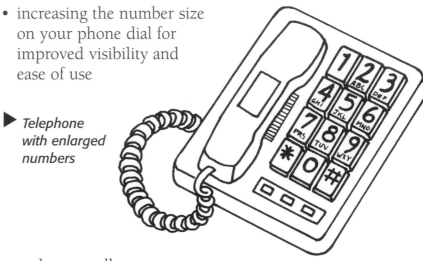

▶ *Telephone with enlarged numbers*

- a phone cradle

- step-by-step, large-size instructions for using the phone

- amplified handsets

- signal devices, such as lights to notify of incoming calls

- TTY (Text Telephone Yoke), a telephone communication device for the hard of hearing

- a portable phone (to keep out of reach of a confused person)

- speed-dial buttons with names or pictures of friends and family instead of numbers

- a one-line phone that automatically connects to a pre-set number when the button is pressed

- a list of emergency numbers and medicines beside the telephone (See *Setting Up a Plan of Care,* page 146, for a sample.)

- clear instructions on how to direct emergency personnel to the street address of the house

- a personal emergency response system to signal a friend or emergency service

 Some communities provide a free Telephone Reassurance Service. There is a brief, daily telephone call to elderly or disabled persons to reassure them and to share crime prevention information. Call your local police department or the Area Agency on Aging.

Outdoor Areas

Safe outdoor areas are important, especially for the frail elderly who are mobile. Safety features should include:

- ramps for access in uneven elevations

- a deck with a sturdy railing

- outside doors locked or alarmed, especially for the person with Alzheimer's

- a hidden key outside

- adequate light to see walkway hazards at night

- non-slip step surfaces in good repair

- stair handrails fastened to their fittings

- step edges marked with reflective paint

- a hedge or fence around the yard and potentially dangerous areas like pools or streams

In addition, disable or remove power tools.

The Home Environment for the Person with **Alzheimer's**

If you are caring for someone with Alzheimer's at home, even temporarily, you are providing a chance for that person to remain in a familiar environment where he or she can build on individual strengths and be encouraged to be as independent as possible. Your goals in adapting the home for this kind of care should be to make it calming and reassuring, safe and supportive.

A safe, comfortable environment can help a person with Alzheimer's feel more relaxed and less overwhelmed. Try to look at the world through that person's eyes and—above all—focus on the prevention of accidents, wandering away from home, and emotional upset.

Safety

- For those who tend to wander, create a safe path through the home for a "wander loop."

- Put reflector tape on furniture and sharp corners

- Place padding on the sharp corners of furniture.

- Use reflector tape to create a path to follow from the bedroom to the bathroom at night.

- Cover radiators with radiator guards.

- Use child-proof plugs in all electrical outlets.

- Lock the cellar and garage doors.

- Lock liquor cabinets.

- Remove all poisonous household items.

- Remove all sharp items.

- Remove poisonous plants from the house and yard.

- Install safety latches/locks on the doors and fenced/gated exteriors. Install alarms on the doors.

- Rid the home of firearms or store them in a locked cabinet, with the bullets in a separate locked cabinet.

- Cover smooth or shiny surfaces to reduce glare, which upsets or confuses the person with Alzheimer's.

- Eliminate shadows by creating a uniform level of light with uplights which reflect off the ceiling. (Ask a lighting store for a lamp that doesn't cast shadows.)

- Cover or remove mirrors if they are upsetting to a person with hallucinations.

- Store car keys in a locked container; disable the car.

- Hide the garage door remote control.

Comfort and Convenience

- Remove items of monetary or sentimental value.

- Lock important documents out of reach.

- Try to have windows low enough to look out when sitting; however, install guards to prevent them from being opened more than 3 inches.

- Choose wall colors that are soothing and are favorites of the person in your care.

The Bathroom

Take great care when setting up the bathroom for the person with Alzheimer's. With some forethought, potential dangers can be averted.

Safety

- Mark the shower wall and faucets with a colored stripe that shows where the temperature should be set.

- Put screens over open drains.

- Put wastebaskets out of sight. (Otherwise, a person with Alzheimer's may urinate in them.)

- Have no electrical cords dangling near the washbasin.

- Remove or lock away all razors and potentially poisonous items.

- Paint hot water faucets red.

- Install an automatic hot and cold water mixer.

- Install faucets that turn off automatically.

- If possible, have the toilet seat and washbasin be in a contrasting color to the floor.

The Kitchen

Kitchen safety is a major issue for Alzheimer's caregivers, who must make every effort to anticipate potential problems. It is always best to remove things if they cause frustration.

Safety

- Remove all items that cause confusion.

- Remove the freezer door handle.

- Put a lock on the refrigerator.

- Disguise the garbage disposal switches.

- Put all the garbage out of sight.

- Put labels on the cabinets.

- Install a shut-off valve (for a gas stove) or a circuit breaker for an electric stove so you can disable it when you leave the kitchen.

- Remove burner knobs and tape the stems or install knob covers.

▶ *For ease of feeding the person with Alzheimer's, use a vinyl desk chair with locking wheels*

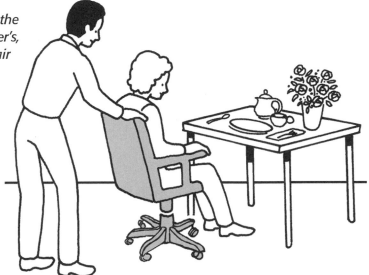

- Use a lock-out switch on the electric range so it can't be turned on except by you.

- Use an aluminum cover over the top of the stove, or use burner covers.

- Replace the pilot on a gas stove with an electric starter.

- Lock the oven door.

- Use safety latches on doors and cabinets.

- Install gates, doors, or dutch doors so the kitchen can be closed off but you can still be seen.

- Install an automatic turn-off on the faucet.

- Install a governor on the hot water faucet (or turn down the valve under the sink) to control the amount of water that can be used.

- For a faucet spout that swings outside the sink itself, install a brace that keeps water in the sink at all times.

- Hide or get rid of dangerous small appliances.

- Turn off appliances by unplugging them, turning off circuit breakers, or removing fuses.

REDUCING MEMORY PROBLEMS

Memory loss can be a severe problem, especially for someone with Alzheimer's, but some everyday steps can be taken to help out.

- Colored paper or a picture of the toilet can be taped on bathroom door.

- Drawers, cabinets, and refrigerators can be labeled.

- Objects can be in contrasting colors so they stand out.

- Notes can be placed in plain sight as reminders of things the person in your care should do.

The Bedroom

Nighttime wandering is a problem that must be considered when setting up a bedroom for a person with Alzheimer's.

Safety

- Place an alarm mat at the side of the bed, use an infrared sensor beam for sounding an alarm when a person crosses it, or attach a monitor to clothing.

▶ *To prevent injuries, attach pillows to the sides of the bed or cover bed rails with water-pipe insulation tubing.*

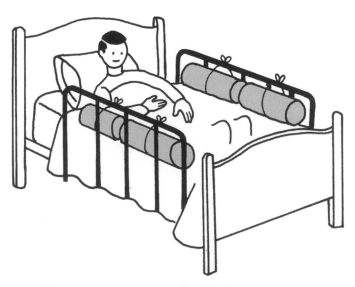

- For anyone who is a wanderer, lower the bed height by removing casters, box springs, or legs; place the dresser at the end of the bed.

- Reverse the headboard and footboard to prevent the person from climbing out of bed—or use bed rails.

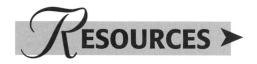

RESOURCES ➤

Area Agency on Aging
Your local Area Agency on Aging provides home safety resources.

Center for Universal Design
North Carolina State University
Box 8613
Raleigh, NC 27695-8613
(919) 515-3082 (V/TTY)
Fax (919) 515-3023
(800) 647-6777
www.design.ncsu.edu\cud
E-mail: cud@ncsu.edu
Established in 1989 by the National Institute on Disability and Rehabilitation Research (NIDRR) to improve the quality and availability of housing for people with disabilities. Services include information, referral service, training and education, technical design assistance, and publications.

AARP
601 E Street, NW
Washington, DC 20049
(800) 424-3410
www.aarp.org
Call or write for the booklet, The Do-Able, Renewable Home. *Members can receive one copy at no charge.*

National Association of Home Builders Research Center
(301) 249-4000
(800) 638-8556
www.nahbrc.org
Call for its book, A Comprehensive Approach to Retrofitting Houses for a Lifetime, *$15 plus postage and handling.*

Check with local police to find out if they manage a **Senior Locks Program.** This is a program whereby homeowners 55 and older who meet federal income guidelines can have dead-bolt locks and other security devices installed for free.

Equipment and Supplies

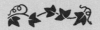

Equipment and Supplies

To provide proper at-home care, you will need to acquire certain supplies, which fall into two categories:

- *general medical supplies*
- *durable medical equipment*

Before buying equipment or signing any contract for rental, consult your doctor, physical or occupational therapist, or nurse. Salespeople may not have training in assessing all medical, social, and environmental factors to make a good decision. Occupational therapists can consult on low-cost substitutes for expensive equipment. With appropriate doctor's orders and documentation, some equipment is covered by Medicare or private insurance. Contact your insurance carrier to check if the equipment is covered and follow the procedure for pre-authorization.

Where to Buy Needed Supplies

Medical equipment and supplies should be purchased from well-established outlets. Seek out dealers with a reputation for good service. Be sure to get recommendations from your health care professionals or hospital discharge planner. To compare prices, use the chart on page 130 as a sample worksheet.

Look in the Yellow Pages under Surgical Appliances, Physicians and Surgeons, Equipment & Supplies, and First Aid Supplies. Outlets include:

- surgical supply stores
- pharmacies

- hospitals
- home health care agencies
- department stores
- medical supply catalogs

Where to Borrow

For short-term use, consider borrowing equipment. Call your local—

- Salvation Army
- Red Cross
- Visiting Nurses Association
- home health care agencies
- National Easter Seal Society
- Muscular Dystrophy Association
- American Cancer Society
- charity organizations
- churches, senior centers, leisure clubs

 Never buy equipment from a telephone solicitor, a door-to-door salesman, or a person who calls on you before the doctor or hospital discharge planner has told you what equipment will be needed.

Checklist *General Supplies*

- ✓ antibacterial hand cleaner
- ✓ bacteriostatic ointment
- ✓ bandages, gauze pads, tape
- ✓ blankets (2–3)
- ✓ cotton balls and swabs
- ✓ toothbrush
- ✓ denture or dental care items
- ✓ kidney-shaped basin for oral care
- ✓ diabetic needle disposal container
- ✓ disposable moisture-repellent Chux underpad for bed protection
- ✓ draw sheets for use in turning someone in bed
- ✓ finger towels for washcloths
- ✓ foam rubber pillows
- ✓ head pillows
- ✓ heating pad
- ✓ hydrogen peroxide
- ✓ ice bag
- ✓ lotion
- ✓ 4 sheets (at least)

- ✓ oral laxative
- ✓ poster with first aid procedures
- ✓ pressure pad and pump
- ✓ rubber sterile gloves
- ✓ rubbing alcohol
- ✓ seat belts (to prevent sliding down in a chair)
- ✓ shower cap
- ✓ soap for dry skin
- ✓ thermometers (rectal and oral)
- ✓ tissues
- ✓ disposable underpants
- ✓ incontinent briefs
- ✓ pants liners
- ✓ toilet paper tongs to take care of personal hygiene
- ✓ waterproof sheeting
- ✓ roll belt restraint
- ✓ gait/transfer belt
- ✓ Medic Alert® identification
- ✓ Safe Return identification bracelet for wanderers (See *Safe Return Program*, page 302.)

How to Pay

Be creative in seeking help in paying for equipment. Consider—

- asking the doctor to write an order for a home evaluation, including an evaluation of needed equipment.

- finding out if the equipment is partially or completely covered by private health insurance with home care benefits.

- checking state retirement and union programs.

Medicare does *not* help pay for assistive devices, but does pay for durable medical equipment in some cases. To qualify for medical coverage, the equipment must be prescribed by a doctor and it must be medically necessary. It must be useful only to a sick or injured person and be able to be used over and over. Medicare will pay for the rental of certain items for no more than 15 months, after which you have the option to buy the equipment from the supplier. If the person in your care has met the deductible, Medicare will pay 80% of the approved charges on the rental, purchase, and service of equipment that the doctor has ordered.

GETTING ORGANIZED

Keep supplies together that are used often and keep a list of supplies so you can easily replace them.

Be prepared for emergencies. Have on hand a flashlight, a battery operated radio, a battery operated clock, fresh batteries, extra blankets, candles with holders, matches, and a manual can opener.

Medical Equipment

You will need to provide special equipment for various rooms in the house, as well as equipment to increase mobility for the person receiving care.

Equipment for the Bedroom

The types of equipment you need to acquire depend on the person's medical condition. This equipment might include some of the items listed below.

- **hospital bed**—allows positioning not possible in a regular bed and aids in resting and breathing more comfortably as well as getting in and out of bed more easily

- **alternating pressure mattress**—minimizes stress on skin tissue from pressure

- **egg carton pad**—a foam mattress pad shaped like an egg carton that reduces pressure and improves air circulation

- **portable commode chair**—for ease of toileting at the bedside

- **trapeze bar**—provides support and a secure hand-hold while changing positions

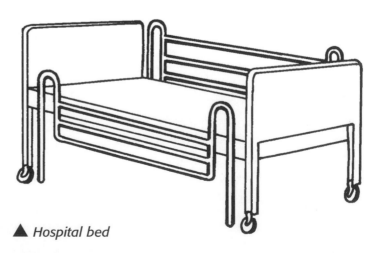

▲ *Hospital bed*

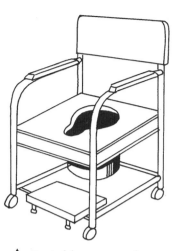

▲ *Portable commode chair*

- **transfer board**—a smooth board for independent or assisted transfer from bed to wheelchair, toilet, or portable commode (📖 See page 284)

- **hydraulic lift**—for use on a difficult to move person

- **over-the-bed table**—provides a surface for activities such as eating, reading, writing, and game playing (could be an adjustable ironing board)

- **mechanical or electric lift chair**—for help getting up from a chair

- **blanket support**—a wire support that keeps heavy bed linens off injured areas or the feet

- **urinal and bed pan**—for toileting in the bed

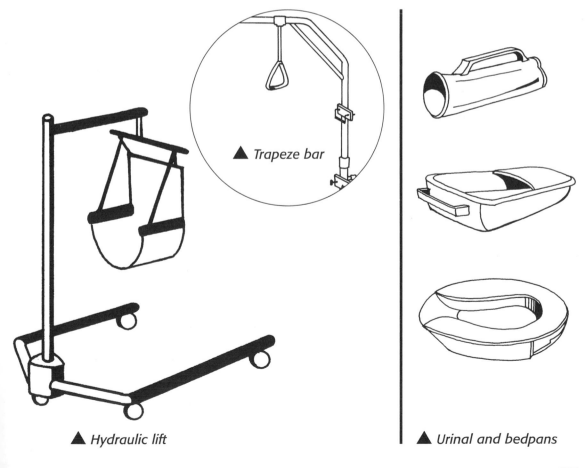

▲ *Trapeze bar*

▲ *Hydraulic lift*

▲ *Urinal and bedpans*

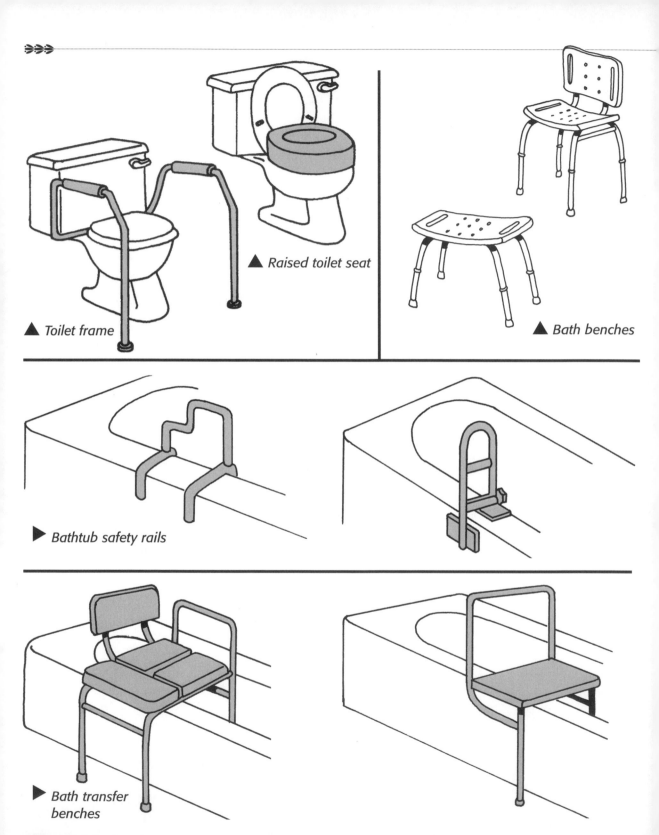

▲ Raised toilet seat

▲ Toilet frame

▲ Bath benches

▶ Bathtub safety rails

▶ Bath transfer benches

Equipment for the Bathroom

Equipment needs depend on individual circumstances. You should consider providing—

- **raised toilet seat**—a seat used to assist a person who has difficulty getting up or down on a toilet (available in molded plastic and clamp-on models for different toilet bowl styles)

- **commode aid**—a device that acts as an elevated toilet seat when used with a splash guard, or as a commode when used with a pail

- **toilet frame**—a free-standing unit that fits over the toilet and provides supports on either side for ease of getting up and down

- **grab bars for tub and shower**—properly installed wall-mounted safety bars that hold a person's weight

- **safety mat and strips**—rough vinyl strips that adhere to the bottom of the tub and shower to prevent slipping

- **hand-held shower hose**—a movable shower hose and head that allows the flow of water to be directed to all parts of the body

- **bath bench**—aid for a person who has difficulty sitting down in or getting up from the bottom of the tub

- **bath transfer bench**—a bench that straddles the side of the tub and allows a person to get out of the tub easily

- **bathtub safety rails**—support for getting in and out of the tub

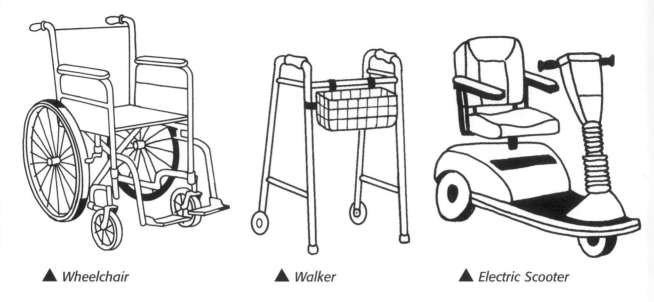

▲ *Wheelchair* ▲ *Walker* ▲ *Electric Scooter*

Mobility Aids

Mobility aids include devices that help a person move around without help, as well as those that help the caregiver manage transfers in and out of bed and from bed to a chair.

They include—

- a wheelchair with padding and removable arms

- a walker to help maintain balance and provide some support

- a 3- or 4-wheel electric scooter

- crutches for use when weight cannot be put on one leg or foot

- a cane to provide light weight-bearing support

- a transfer board (9" x 24") for moving someone in and out of bed (📖 See illustration page 284.)

- a gait/transfer belt (📖 See illustration of use on page 281.)

▼ *Canes*

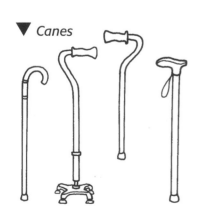

MOBILITY

A baby stroller helps a person maintain balance, provides some support, is easy to move from room to room, and provides a large surface for carrying items from room to room.

Wheelchair Requirements

- safety
- durability
- ease of repair
- attractive appearance

- comfort
- ease of maneuvering
- cushions

USING CANES

Attach Velcro® to the top of a cane and a piece of Velcro® to counters and bedside tables to keep the cane from falling when not in use.

Wheelchair Attachments for Stroke Patients

- a brake extension
- elevated leg and removable foot rests
- removable arm rests

 Some states have enacted "lemon" laws covering wheelchairs and other assistive devices. If you think the equipment you have bought is defective and you want to determine if it qualifies as a "lemon", contact the Attorney General's office in your state for guidance in getting a replacement or a refund.

Specialized Equipment

For those with poor sight, hearing, and other limitations, many aids exist to make life easier. Explore all the options and you will find that your job as caregiver becomes easier too.

Sight Aids

- prism glasses

- magnifying glasses

- prescription glasses

- Braille books and signs

- cassette players and books on tape

- telesensory devices that convert printed letters into symbols that can be touched

Listening Aids

- hearing aids (order from an audiologist who allows a free 30-day trial and is a registered dealer)

- sound amplification systems

- telephone amplifiers

- devices that make it possible to receive close-captioned TV programs

HELP FOR SPECIAL EQUIPMENT
Tip
Investigate whether Medicaid or Lion's Clubs in your state can pay for hearing aids.

Eating Aids

- swivel spoons for those who have trouble with wrist movement

- cylindrical foam that enlarges gripping surfaces so utensils can be lifted more easily

- plate guards or high-sided dishes that make it easier to scoop food onto a spoon

- rocker knives that can cut food with a rocking motion

- food-warming dishes for slow eaters

- mugs with two handles, covers, spouts, and suction bases

▼ *Eating aids—mug, built-up handles, food guard, one hand knife, swivel spoon*

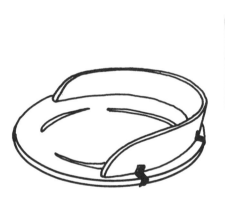
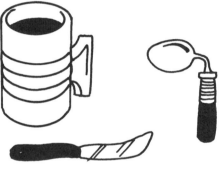

Dressing Aids

- button hooks that make buttoning clothes easy

- dressing sticks that make it possible to dress without bending

- shoe horns that eliminate the need to bend over when putting on shoes

- sock aids that keep stockings open while they are being put on

(📖 See examples on next page.)

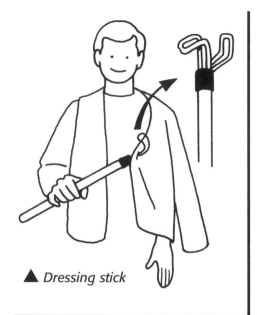

▲ Dressing stick

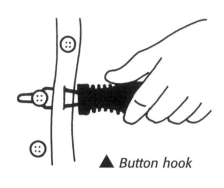

▲ Button hook

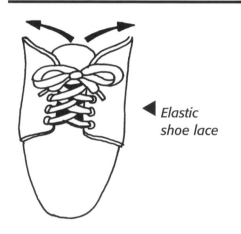

◀ Elastic
shoe lace

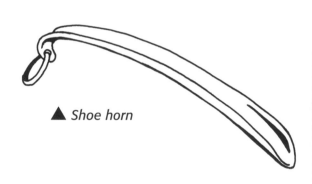

▲ Shoe horn

Tip

PUTTING ON SHOES

For people who have difficulty tying laces, turn a lace-up shoe into a slip-on shoe by replacing the cotton shoelaces with elastic ones.

Devices for Summoning Help

- touch-tone phones with speed dials

- wireless transmitters for emergency response

- medical security response systems

- beepers for the caregiver

Homemade Aids and Gadgets

- wrist straps for canes—tape tied on a cane so it can be hung from the wrist while walking upstairs

- kitchen chair trolleys—made by putting castors on a chair so things placed on the seat can be moved

- bicycle baskets—strapped to a walker to store necessities and free hands

- an egg carton—to organize pills

- rubber safety-mats—ideal for the tub, shower, or anywhere the feet can slip; also useful to make non-slip surfaces on trays and tables

- key enlargements—made by putting a key into a large cork

- foot-operated door levers—made by attaching rope to a "stirrup" and tying it to the lever handle

- enlarged handles—handlebar-style grips made with a garden hose, bendable aluminum tubing, a paint roller cover, or (on small surfaces) a foam hair curler roller

- language tags—cardboard tags with words that can be used to express needs

- light switch enlargements—made by putting a rubber pen cap over a light switch

- enlarged pull switches—made by putting a plastic ball over small switches

- clips for canes—spring clips or Velcro® placed on favorite chairs to keep a cane from falling

- bedside rails—wooden rails attached to the floor at right angles on swivel hinges

- pull rope—rope attached to the foot board of the bed to help someone change positions in bed

Equipment Cost Comparison Chart *(Example)*

Items	Purchase Price	Rental Fee × Months Needed	Covered by Medicare Yes/No
bath stool	$		
bed pan			
bed safety accessories			
cane			
commode			
crutches			
hospital bed			
mattress			
oxygen			
raised toilet seat			
special equipment			
trapeze			
walker			
wheelchair			
3- or 4-wheel scooter			
other			
Totals	$		

Specialized Hospital-Type Equipment

- **oxygen tanks,** for use when oxygen is needed as a medication

- **transtracheal oxygen therapy equipment,** for use when oxygen is delivered into the lungs through a flexible tube that goes from the neck directly into the trachea

- **compressors and hand-held nebulizers,** which reduce medication to a form that can be inhaled

- **suction catheters,** which clear mucus and secretions from the back of the throat when someone cannot swallow

- **home infusion equipment,** or intravenous (IV) therapy, which delivers antibiotics, blood products, chemotherapy, hydration, pain management, parenteral (IV) nutrition, and specialty medications

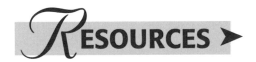

RESOURCES ➤

Sears Home Health Care Catalogue
(800) 326-1750 for Customer Service
To place an order or find a Sears store near you.

Sammons-Preston
Bowling Brook, IL
(800) 323-5547

NCM Aftertherapy Catalog
(800) 235-7054

Lumex
(800) 645-5272

Briggs
(800) 247-2343

Lighthouse International for the Blind
111 E 59th Street
New York, NY 10022
(212) 821-9200
(800) 829-0500
www.lighthouse.org
Provides free information on eye-related diseases and can refer individuals to resources in your community. Has a free catalog on low-vision aides.

Abledata
8630 Fenton Street, Suite 930
Silver Spring, MD 20910-3319
(800) 227-0216
(301) 608-8998
Fax (301) 608-8958
www.abledata.com
Stores information on thousands of assistive devices for home health care, from eating utensils to wheelchairs. Provides prices, names, and addresses of suppliers.

American Occupational Therapy Association (AOTA)
4720 Montgomery Lane
P.O. Box 31220
Bethesda, MD 20824-1220
(301) 652-2682
Fax (301) 652-7711
www.aota.org
Provides consumer publications.

University of Minnesota Extension Service/Martin County
Extension Educator
Rm. 104 Courthouse
201 Lake Avenue
Fairmount, MN 56031
(800) 967-3340
(507) 235-3341

Fax (507) 235-5772
E-mail: rabbe001@umn.edu
Provides a video on clothing adaptations for elderly with physical limitations for $20 and free educational materials.

Oklahoma State University

Janice M. Park, PhD
Cooperative Extension Service—Family Community Sciences
239340 Human Environmental Sciences
Stillwater, OK 74078
(405) 744-8489 6825
Fax (405) 744-1461 7113
Provides free information for caregivers of the elderly on various topics such as memory, depression and financial planning.

Buffalo State College

Center for Clothing for Individuals with Physical Disabilities
1300 Elmwood Avenue, Caudell Hall 301
Buffalo, NY 14222-1095
(716) 878-5813
Fax (716) 878-30335834
Provides a list of clothing manufacturers specializing in adaptable clothing including sizes, color and cost for $5, includingplus shipping and handling. Also provides written information regarding sewing patterns and ready-to-wear clothing modifications for a nominal fee.

AT&T Special Needs Center

(800) 872-3883 (TTY)
Provides free directory assistance (with an application) and operator's help dialing for the vision impaired and disabled.

Self Help for Hard of Hearing People (SHHH)
7910 Woodmont Avenue, Suite 1200
Bethesda, MD 20814
(301) 657-2248
(301) 657-2249 (TTY)
Offers information on coping with hearing loss and on hearing aids.

Radio Shack
Carries a variety of alerting devices in stores nationwide.

Medic Alert®
(800) 432-5378
Offers critically important medical facts about the emblem wearer's condition to emergency personnel 24 hours a day.

For **medical alarms,** consult the phone book or contact your local hospital's long-term care or senior services division.

The Alzheimers Store
www.thealzheimersstore.com
Provides information and unique products for caregivers of someone with Alzheimers.

Part Two: Day by Day

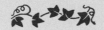

Part 2 ✥ Day by Day

Setting Up a Plan of Care

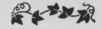

Setting Up a Plan of Care

A Plan of Care is a daily record of the care and treatment a person needs after a hospital stay. The Plan helps you and anyone who assists you with caregiving tasks.

When a patient leaves a hospital, the discharge planner provides the caregiver with a copy of the doctor's orders and a brief set of instructions for care. The discharge planner also arranges for a home health care agency to send a nurse, who will evaluate the patient's needs for equipment, personal care, help with shots or medication, etc. The nurse will also work with the entire health care team (including you, the caregiver, a physical therapist, and other specialists) to develop a detailed Plan of Care.

The Plan of Care includes the following information:

- diagnosis

- medications

- functional limitations

- a list of equipment needed

- specific diet

- detailed care instructions and comments

- services the home health care agency provides

This information is presented in a specific order so that the process of care becomes repetitive and routine. When the Plan is kept up to date, it provides a clear record of events that is helpful both in solving and in avoiding problems.

The Plan also keeps you from having to rely on your memory and allows another person to take over respite care or take your place entirely with a minimum of disruption.

Some of the things you may have to observe and record are:

- skin color, warmth, and tone (dryness, firmness, etc.)
- pressure areas where bed sores can develop (See *Activities of Daily Living,* page 188.)
- breathing, temperature, pulse, and blood pressure
- circulation (dark red or blue spots on the legs or feet)
- finger and toe nails (any unusual conditions)
- mobility
- puffiness around the eyes and cheeks, swelling of the hands and ankles
- appetite
- body posture (relaxed, twisted, or stiff)
- bowel and bladder function (unusual changes)

Recording the Plan of Care

To record the Plan of Care, use a loose-leaf notebook. Put the doctor's instructions on the inside front cover (always keep the originals). Include in the notebook the types of forms that appear in the following pages in this chapter. These pages should be three-hole punched.

After using your Plan of Care for one week, make necessary adjustments and continue to do so as the person's needs change. Always adjust to what works for you and the person being cared for. Use notes, pictures, or whatever it takes to describe your responsibilities. Also, use black ink, not pencil, to maintain a permanent record.

Daily Activities Record (Sample Form)

Day/Date: _____

Morning _____

_____

Afternoon _____

_____

Naps: Time _____ Place _____

Evening _____

Activities	Yes	No	Where/How/When
Walk	☐	☐	_____
TV	☐	☐	_____
Reading Aloud	☐	☐	_____
Visitors	☐	☐	_____
Calls to Friends/Relatives	☐	☐	_____
Other			

Bedtime Routine	Yes	No	Where/How
Incontinence Pad/Brief	☐	☐	_____
Medication	☐	☐	_____
Special Pillow/Blanket	☐	☐	_____
Music/Radio/TV	☐	☐	_____
Nightlight	☐	☐	_____
Restraints, Calming Techniques	☐	☐	_____
Urinal/Bedpan	☐	☐	_____
Gates at Doors/on Stairs	☐	☐	_____
Oral/Denture Care	☐	☐	_____
Foot Care	☐	☐	_____

Braces ☐   Fungus ☐   Massage ☐   Ingrown Nails ☐   Nail Care ☐

Meals

Help Needed with Meals _____

Meal Times _____

Special Diet _____

Foods to Avoid _____

Special Utensils _____

Snacks _____

Favorite Foods _____

Location of Meals _____

Daily Care Record (Sample Form)   Day/Date: _____

Daily Activities/Limitations:

Walks Alone_____ Stands Alone _____

Bed Position_____

Equipment Used: Walker ☐   Cane ☐   Wheelchair ☐   Brace ☐

How long _____

ROM/Exercises: Upper Body ☐   Lower Body ☐   Goes Outside ☐

Meals: Special Diet ☐

Breakfast _____

Lunch _____

Dinner _____

Snack _____

Fluids _____

Treatments

Catheter _____

Oxygen _____

Equipment _____

Physical Therapy _____

Special Precautions _____

Resuscitate ☐   Do Not Resuscitate ☐

Personal Care

Bath: ☐ Bed   ☐ Chair

Shower: ☐ Tub   ☐ Bench

Care of Genitals: _____

Nail Care: ☐ Toes   ☐ Fingers

Oral Care: ☐ Brush Teeth   ☐ Floss Teeth   ☐ Dentures

Hair Care: ☐ Shave   ☐ Bed Shampoo   ☐ Bath/Shampoo

Skin Care: ☐ Lotion Upper Body   ☐ Lotion Lower Body   ☐ Powdered

Massage: ☐ Head and Shoulder   ☐ Leg and Foot   ☐ Back

Bowel Movements _____ Voiding _____ Quantity _____

Temperature _____ Blood Pressure _____ Respiration _____

Comments/Attitudes/Conditions   _____

_____

_____

Visitors   _____

_____

Activities Schedule for Backup Caregiver (Sample Form)

Personal Needs	Yes	No	Where to Find
Cane	☐	☐	_____
Dentures	☐	☐	_____
Glasses	☐	☐	_____
Hearing aid	☐	☐	_____
Walker	☐	☐	_____

Morning Routine

Breakfast _____ Where Eaten _____

Amount of Help Needed _____

Special Utensils Needed _____

Medications with Meals ☐ _____ Nap ☐ _____

Snack Foods _____ Time of Snack _____

Evening Routine

Dinner _____ Where Eaten _____

Evening Snack _____

Bedtime Routine

Help Needed Undressing ☐ _____ Shower or Bath Needed ☐

Where Clothes Are Stored _____

Where Dentures Are Stored _____

Special Items Needed: _____

Incontinent Pad/Brief ☐ _____ Urinal ☐ _____ Restraints ☐

Special Pillows ☐ _____ Music ☐ _____ Nightlight ☐

Calming Techniques _____

_____

Special Concerns or Equipment

Catheter ☐ _____ Oxygen ☐ _____

Special Precautions _____

Other _____

Resuscitate ☐　　　**Do Not Resuscitate ☐**

Be on the Alert for:

Wandering _____

Gates on Stairs/Locks on Doors _____

Alarms _____

Other _____

Don't be surprised if: _____

Recording and Managing Medications

People who have serious health problems often take a large number of medications at many different times of the day. It is essential to have a careful system for keeping track of—

- when medications should be given

- how they should be administered

- when were they actually given

The following sample Weekly Medication Schedule is a good model to follow. Be sure to fill in the times when (A.M. and P.M.) medications actually were given, and have each caregiver initial them.

Weekly Medication Schedule (Sample Form)

Medication	Date/Time/Initials						
Name, dose, frequency, with food, without food	Sat.	Sun.	Mon.	Tues.	Wed.	Thurs.	Fri.
Example							
2 mg. Coumadin 1x daily am with food	8:30am	8:00am	9:00am	8:45am	9:00am	8:30am	7:45am
400 mg. folic acid 1x daily am	8:30am	8:00am	9:00am	8:45am	9:00am	8:30am	7:45am
Fruitlax 1 Tbsp. evening only	6pm	6pm	6:30pm	6:45pm	6:15pm	6:30pm	7:00pm
Visine	10am	10am		4pm			

As you complete your own schedule, be sure to record information from the label of each prescription, including—

• days of the week when each medicine must be taken

• number of times per day

• time of day

• whether the medicine is to be taken with or without food

• how much water should be taken with the medicine

Also make a note to yourself about—

• any warnings (for example, "Don't take this medicine with alcohol.")

• possible side effects (dizziness, confusion, headache, etc.)

NOTE Labels may contain the following abbreviations, so be aware of their meanings—

HS-Hour of Sleep (medication time)
BID-give the medicine 2 times per day (approximately 8 and 8)
TID-give the medicine 3 times per day (approximately 9-1-6)
QID-give the medicine 4 times per day (approximately 9-1-5-9)

Some Other Cautions

• Never crush drugs without consulting the doctor or pharmacist. If the person in your care has difficulty swallowing medication, ask the doctor for another way to administer it. (See *Using the Health Care Team Effectively,* page 26.)

• If the person in your care will take the medicine without your oversight, ask the pharmacist to prepackage dosages or devise a color code for multiple medications.

- Do not store medicine for internal and external use in the same cabinet.

- Keep a magnifying glass near the medicine cabinet.

- Store most medicine in a cool, dry place—usually not the bathroom.

- Remove the cotton from each bottle so that moisture is not drawn in.

- Flush all medicine not currently being used down the toilet.

- Ask the pharmacist for non-child proof containers if the child-proof ones are too hard to open.

Tip

EMERGENCY PREPAREDNESS
Notify the local fire station and ambulance company that a disabled person lives at this address. They will have the information on hand and can respond quickly.

Emergency Information

Have this information posted near telephones or on the refrigerator, where it can be used by anyone in the household in case of emergency.

Personal Information

Name _____ Date of Birth _____

Address _____

Phone _____

SS # _____ Supplemental Insurance # _____

Medicaid # _____ Medicare # _____

Current Medications: _____

_____

Exact Location of Do Not Resuscitate Order: _____

Emergency Numbers

Fire _____ Police _____

Ambulance _____ Hospital _____

Doctor _____

Alzheimer's Association's Safe Return Hotline _____

Drugstore _____ Open Till _____ Delivers _____

Family Caregiver Work Number _____

Alternate Caregiver _____

Home Health Care Agency _____

Medicare Toll Free Number _____

Insurance _____

Medical Equipment Company _____

Poison Control _____

Friend _____

_____

Neighbor _____ Relative _____

Clergy/Rabbi _____

Transport Number _____ Meals-on-Wheels _____

Shopping Assistance _____

_____

Directions for Driving to the House _____

_____

_____

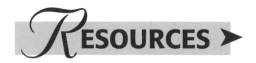
RESOURCES ➤

Elder Health Program
Peter Lamy Center on Drug Therapy and Aging
School of Pharmacy
University of Maryland at Baltimore
506 West Fayette Street
Room 106
Baltimore, MD 21201
(410) 706-2434
Fax: (410) 706-1488
www.pharmacy.umaryland.edu/lamy
Provides free information about older people and medications.

How to Avoid Caregiver Burnout

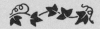

How to Avoid Caregiver Burnout

*B*urnout, the complete drain of our physical, spiritual, and emotional reserves, occurs when a caregiver slips beyond exhaustion or depression. Every day, caregivers face the need to remove themselves emotionally from their task or risk entering so deeply into it that they burn out. Anyone who cares for a person whose health is deteriorating needs understanding, support, and help—from friends, family, and a support group.

As primary caregiver, your most important duty is to conserve your strength and restore your resources. Remember, you are the one who is going to make it all happen over the long term, so guard your health!

Emotional Burdens You Face

You may have thought that the following problems were unique to your situation, but they are not. Every caregiver faces:

- the need to hide grief

- fear of the future

- worry about finances

- lessened ability to solve problems

NOTE Men who undertake caregiving face special problems because often they are not familiar with everyday homemaking chores. Additionally, they lose the emotional support of the spouse who is ill and must now be *her* support. It is especially important for men to seek out support groups.

Knowing When to Seek Help

If you have been a caregiver for an extended period and have great difficulty with the stressful situation, seek professional counseling through a home health care agency, the local American Red Cross, or your religious service agency.

You need professional help with the burden when you:

- are using more and more alcohol to relax

- are using too many prescription medications

- have physical symptoms such as skin rashes, backaches, or a lingering cold or flu

- feel unable to concentrate

- feel lethargic

- feel keyed up and on edge

- feel constant sadness

- feel intense fear and anxiety

- feel worthless and guilty

- are depressed for two weeks or more

- are having thoughts of suicide

- are thinking about becoming or have become physically violent against the person you are caring for

When Hostility Builds to a Breaking Point

You can control your emotions by releasing anger and frustration in a safe way.

- Take a walk to cool down.

- Write your thoughts in a journal.

- Go to a private corner and unleash your anger on a big pillow.

Where to Find Professional Help or Support-Group Counseling

- the community pages of the phone directory
- the local county medical society, which can provide a list of counselors, psychologists, and psychiatrists

Checklist **Dealing with Physical and Emotional Burdens**

✓ *Do not allow the person in your care to take unfair advantage of you by being overly demanding.*

✓ *Live one day at a time.*

✓ *List priorities, decide what to leave undone, and think of ways to streamline the work.*

✓ *When doing a long, boring care task, use the time to relax or listen to music.*

✓ *Find time for regular exercise to increase your energy (even if you can only stretch in place).*

✓ *Concentrate on getting relaxed sleep rather than more sleep.*

✓ *Take several short rests to get adequate sleep.*

✓ *Set aside time for prayer and reflection.*

✓ *Practice deep breathing and learn to meditate to empty your mind of all troubles.*

✓ *Allow your self-esteem to rise because you have discovered hidden skills and talents.*

✓ *Realize your own limitations and accept them.*

✓ *Make sure your goals are realistic—you may be unable to do everything you could before.*

✓ *Keep your nutrition balanced—do not fall into a toast-and-tea habit.*

- religious service agencies

- community health clinics

- clergy or rabbi

- Area Agency on Aging

✓ *Claim time for yourself.*

✓ *Treat yourself to a massage.*

✓ *Keep up with outside friends and activities.*

✓ *Spread the word that help will be gratefully received, and allow friends to help with respite care.*

✓ *Delegate jobs to others. Keep a list of tasks you need to have done and assign specific ones when people offer to help.*

✓ *Share your concerns and dilemmas with a friend.*

✓ *Join a support group, or start one (to share ideas and resources).*

✓ *Use respite care when needed.*

✓ *Communicate openly and honestly with people whom you feel should do more to help.*

✓ *When you visit your own doctor, be sure to explain your caregiving responsibilities, not just your symptoms.*

✓ *Allow yourself to feel the emotions you feel without guilt. They are natural and very human.*

✓ *Unload your anger and frustration by writing it down.*

✓ *Let yourself cry and sob.*

✓ *Know that you are providing a very important service to someone you love.*

- United Way's "First Call for Help"

- a hospital's social service department

- a newspaper calendar listing of support group meetings

- parish nurses

Ask a counselor familiar with the needs of caregivers.

How to Let Friends Help You

If your friends want to know how they can help ease your burden, tell them to:

- telephone and be a good listener as you may voice strong feelings

- offer words of appreciation for your efforts

- share a meal

- help you find useful information about community resources

- show genuine interest

- stop by or send cards, letters, pictures, or humorous newspaper clippings

- share the workload

- help hire a relief caregiver

Help you remember the saying, "Grant me the serenity to accept the things I cannot change, the courage to change the things I can, and the wisdom to know the difference."

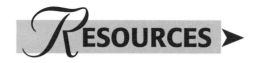

RESOURCES ►

CAPS (Children of Aging Parents)
1609 Woodbourne Road, Suite 302A
Levittown, PA 19057-1511
(800) 227-7294
www.caps4caregivers.org
A nonprofit organization of caregiver support with groups, resources, and information.

Caregiver Survival Resources
www.caregiver911.com
A comprehensive list linking caregiving information and services for general issues and specific chronic illnesses.

Eldercare Locator
(800) 677-1116
www.eldercare.gov
Finds adult protective services in your area for someone experiencing domestic violence. Locates other local resources providing services to the elderly.

Well Spouse Foundation
30 E. 40th St., Penthouse
New York, NY 10016
(800) 838-0879
(212) 685-8815
Fax (212) 685-8676
www.wellspouse.org
E-mail: wellspouse@aol.com
Has a bi-monthly newsletter written by and for well spouses, offers local support groups for well spouses, and provides pamphlets that address the needs of well spouses.

National Family Caregivers Association
10400 Connecticut Avenue, Suite 500
Kensington, MD. 20895-2504
(800) 896-3650
(301) 942-6430
Fax (301) 942-2302
info@nfcacares.org
www.nfcacares.org
Publishes a member newsletter at no charge for family caregivers. Dues are $40 for professionals, $60 for non-profits, and $100 for for-profit organizations.

Center for Family Caregivers/Tad Publishing Co.
(847) 823-0639
www.caregiving.com or www.familycaregivers.org
Develop and distribute educational materials on caregiving, including a newsletter. Caregiving informational kits are $5 each; please specify new, seasoned and transitioning caregiver when requesting a kit.

Check with your local church or health facility to see if they sponsor **"Share the Care"** teams.

If you don't have home access to the Internet, ask your local library to help you locate any Web site.

Activities of Daily Living

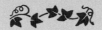

Activities of Daily Living

Personal Hygiene

As a caregiver, you will find that some of your time each day will be devoted to assisting the person in your care with personal hygiene. This includes bathing, shampooing, oral or mouth care, shaving, and foot care.

The Bed Bath

Bed baths are needed by patients who are bedridden. Baths clean, stimulate, and increase circulation in the skin, but they can also dry skin and—in some instances—cause chapping. Thus, you must decide how often a bed bath is needed, and your decision must be based on the particular situation of the person in your care. (If urinary incontinence, bowel problems, and heavy perspiration are present, for example, a daily bath may be in order. If not, bathing 2–3 times a week might be enough.) Make it a habit to use the bath as a time to examine the whole body for bedsores, edema, rash, moles, and other unusual conditions. If baths are given often and the skin is dry, use soap and water one time and lotion and water the next. Cornstarch and powder can cause skin problems in some people. Ask your nurse for advice.

Tip

SKIN CARE
It is easier to prevent chapping than to heal chapped skin, so apply lotion often.

To avoid spreading of germs, always wash your own hands before and after giving a bath. Be aware that the elderly are often afraid of water. Tell the person that you will be bathing him, and ask for as much help as possible. At each step, tell the person what you are about to do.

1. Make sure the room is warm.

2. Gather supplies—latex gloves, mild soap, washcloth, wash basin, lotion, comb, electric razor, shampoo—and clean clothes.

3. Use good body mechanics—keep your feet separated, stand firmly, bend your knees, and keep your back in neutral. (See page 268.)

4. Offer the bedpan or urinal.

5. If possible, raise the bed level to its highest position and bring the head of the bed to an upright position.

6. Help with oral hygiene—brushing the teeth or cleansing the mouth. (See page 168.)

7. Test the water in the basin with your hand.

8. Remove the person's clothes, the blanket, and the top sheet; cover the person with a towel or light blanket. Keep all of the body covered during the bed bath, uncovering only one area at a time while washing it.

9. Now have the person lie almost flat.

10. Have one washcloth for soap, one for rinsing, and a dry towel. Have the washcloth very damp, but not dripping.

11. Very gently wash the face first; pat dry.

NOTE Always wash from the cleanest to the dirtiest.

12. Wash the front of the neck; pat dry.

13. Wash the chest and for females, under the breasts; pat dry.

14. Wash the abdomen, upper thighs; pat dry.

15. Clean the navel with a little lotion on a cotton swab.

16. Wash upward from wrist to upper arm to stimulate circulation; pat dry.

17. Wash the hands and between the fingers; check the nails; pat dry.

18. Place a towel under the person's buttocks.

19. Flex the knees.

20. Wash the legs; pat dry.

21. Wash the feet and between the toes and dry well. Use lotion on dry feet. Do not put lotion between toes. This area must be kept dry and clean to prevent fungal infection.

22. Wash the pubic area. If possible, have the person wash his or her own genitals; if not, do it yourself. (Use PeriWash to prevent bacterial build-up.)

23. If a male is uncircumcised, retract the foreskin, rinse, dry, and bring the foreskin down over the head of the penis again. For the female, wash the genitals thoroughly by spreading the external folds. (This must be done at least daily.)

24. Pat the genitals dry.

25. Watch for unusual tenderness, swelling, or hardness in the testicles.

26. Change the bath water.

27. Roll the person away from you.

28. Tuck a towel under him or her.

29. Wash the back from the neck to the buttocks.

30. Rinse; dry well.

31. Give a back rub with lotion to enhance circulation.

32. Dress the person.

33. Change the bed linens.

34. Trim the toenails if they are long.

 NOTE A build-up of earwax in a bedridden person may obstruct hearing. Have the ears checked and cleaned by a nurse or doctor twice a year. If the doctor approves, apply a little lotion to the outside of the ears to prevent drying and itching.

The Basin Bath

If the person in your care can be in a chair or wheelchair, you can give a sponge bath at the sink.

1. Make sure the room is warm.

2. Gather supplies—latex gloves, mild soap, washcloth, wash basin, lotion, comb, electric razor, shampoo—and clean clothes.

3. Use good body mechanics—keep your feet separated, stand firmly, bend your knees, and keep your back in neutral.

4. Offer the urinal.

5. Wash the face first.

6. Wash the rest of the upper body.

7. If the person can stand, wash the genitals. If the person is too weak to stand, wash the lower part of the body in the bed.

The Tub Bath

If the person in your care has good mobility and is strong enough to get in and out of the tub, he or she may enjoy a tub bath. Be sure there are grab bars, a bath bench, and a rubber mat so the person doesn't slide. (It may be easier to sit at bench level rather than at the bottom of the tub.) Use the following procedure:

1. Make sure the room is warm.

2. Gather supplies—latex gloves for the caregiver, mild soap, washcloth, lotion, comb, electric razor, shampoo—and clean clothes.

3. Check the water temperature before the person gets in.

4. Guide the person into the tub. Have him use the grab bars. (Don't let him grab you and pull you down.)

5. Help the person wash.

6. Empty the tub and then help him get out.

7. Guide the person to use the grab bars while getting out OR have him stand, lower himself onto the bath bench, and swing first one leg, then the other leg, over the edge. Help him stand.

8. Put a towel on a chair or the toilet lid and have the person sit there to dry off.

9. Apply lotion to any skin that appears dry.

10. Help the person dress.

BATHING IN THE TUB
If a bath bench is not used, many people feel more secure if they roll over on to their side and then get on their knees before rising from the tub. It gives them leverage if they are unstable.

The Shower Bath

Remember that the elderly, especially those suffering from Alzheimer's, are often frightened by water. Let the person smell the soap and feel the towel to help him understand. Be sure the shower floor is not slippery.

1. Make sure the room is warm.

2. Explain to the person what you are going to do.

3. Provide a shower stool in case he needs to sit.

4. Gather supplies—mild soap, washcloth, wash basin, comb, electric razor, shampoo—and clean clothes.

5. Turn on the cold water and then the hot to prevent burns. Adjust the water temperature before he gets in and use gentle water pressure.

6. First, spray and clean the less sensitive parts of the body such as the feet.

7. For safety, ask him to hold the grab bar or sit on the shower stool.

8. Move the water hose around the person rather than asking him to move around.

9. Assist in washing as needed.

10. Guide him out of the shower and wrap him in a towel; then turn the water off.

11. Apply lotion to skin that appears dry.

12. If necessary, have him sit on a stool or on the toilet lid.

13. Assist in drying and dressing.

> **NOTE** Remove all electrical equipment that could get wet.

Nail Care

When providing nail care, you can watch for signs of irritation or infection. This is especially important in the diabetic, for whom a small infection can develop into a serious complication. Finger and toe nails can thicken with age, making them more difficult to trim.

1. Assemble supplies—soap, basin with water, towel, nail brush, scissors, nail clippers, file, and lotion.

2. Wash your hands.

3. Wash her hands with soap and water and soak in the basin of warm water for five minutes.

4. Gently scrub the nails with the brush to remove trapped dirt.

5. Dry the nails and gently push back the cuticle with the towel.

6. To prevent ingrown nails, only cut finger and toe nails straight across.

7. File gently to smooth the edges.

8. Gently massage hands and feet with lotion.

 NOTE If other members of the household are using the same equipment, clean the nail clippers with alcohol.

Shampooing the Hair

As people age, they may have difficulty in shampooing their own hair in the shower. Keeping the hair and scalp clean improves circulation to the scalp and keeps the hair healthy. Women especially may consider it a special treat to have their hair styled, but don't be surprised if a person who always enjoyed having her hair done suddenly becomes fearful or reluctant to go through the process. Shampooing can be done anytime the person in your care is not overly tired. Before a bath may be the most convenient time. Adopt a system that is easiest for you and the person in your care.

SHAMPOOING
To make washing easy, dilute the shampoo in a bottle before pouring it on the hair.

Wet Shampoo

1. Assemble supplies—latex gloves, comb and brush, shampoo/conditioner, several pitchers of warm water, large basin, washcloth, towels.

2. Have the person sit on a chair or commode.

3. Drape a large towel over the shoulders.

4. Gently comb knots out of the hair.

5. Protect the person's ears with cotton.

6. Ask her to cover her eyes with a washcloth and to lean over the sink.

7. Moisten the hair with a wet wash cloth or with water poured from a pitcher.

8. Massage a small amount of diluted shampoo into the hair.

9. Remove the shampoo with clean water or a washcloth until the water runs clear when the cloth is wrung out.

10. Use non-rinsing conditioner if desired.

11. Towel the hair dry.

12. Remove the cotton from the ears.

13. Comb the hair gently.

14. If desired, use a hair dryer on the cool setting to dry hair, being very careful not to burn the scalp.

   OR

1. Adapt a heavy rubber dish-draining mat by cutting a round slit at the raised edge so that the end can tuck under the person's neck and the water can drain down into the sink.

2. Seat her at the kitchen sink with her back to the mat.

3. Place a towel on her shoulders and place the rubber dish-draining mat with the round cut against the neck and the smooth edge draining into the sink (beauty salon style).

4. Follow the procedure above, using the sink hose or a pitcher to wash and rinse the hair.

Dry Shampoo

1. Assemble supplies—latex gloves for the caregiver, comb and brush, waterless shampoo, and towels.

2. Lather the head until all foam disappears.

3. Towel the hair dry and gently comb it.

 You can buy a waterless shampoo from the pharmacy or at a medical supply company.

Wet Shampoo in Bed

1. Assemble supplies—latex gloves, comb and brush, shampoo/conditioner, several pitchers of warm water, a large basin, plastic sheet, washcloth, towels, and hair dryer.

2. If possible, raise the bed.

3. Help the person lie flat.

4. Protect the bedding with plastic under the head and shoulders.

5. Roll the edges of the plastic inward so the water will run down into a basin placed on a chair next to the head of the bed.

6. Drape a towel over the shoulders.

7. Protect the person's ears with cotton.

8. Cover the person's eyes with a washcloth.

9. Moisten the hair with a wet washcloth.

10. Massage a small amount of diluted shampoo into the hair.

11. Remove the shampoo with a wet washcloth until the water runs clear when the cloth is wrung out.

12. Use non-rinsing conditioner if desired.

13. Towel the hair dry.

14. Remove the cotton from the ears.

15. Comb the hair gently.

16. Use a hair dryer on the cool setting to dry hair, being very careful not to burn the scalp.

EASIER SHAMPOOING

An enema bag attached to an IV pole provides an easy hose for shampooing.

Shaving

Shaving can be done by the person in your care, or you can shave his whiskers with a safety razor or an electric razor. If he wears dentures, make sure they are in his mouth.

1. Assemble supplies—latex gloves, safety razor, shaving cream, washcloth, towel, lotion.

2. Wash your hands.

3. Adjust the light so can you clearly see his face but so that it does not shine in his eyes.

4. Spread a towel under his chin.

5. Soften the beard by wetting the face with a warm, damp washcloth.

6. Apply shaving cream to his face, carefully avoiding the eyes.

7. Hold the skin tight with one hand and using short firm strokes shave in the direction the hair grows.

8. Be careful of sensitive areas.

9. Rinse his skin with a wet washcloth.

10. Pat his face dry with the towel.

11. Apply lotion if the skin appears dry.

NOTE > Never use an electric razor if the person is receiving oxygen.

Oral Care

Oral care includes cleansing the mouth and gums and the teeth or dentures. Daily dental hygiene is important and can cause anxiety in some elderly people. Always be patient and explain what you are about to do. (The person who refuses to brush his teeth can swish and spit out a fluoridated mouthwash rinse.)

1. Gather supplies—latex gloves, a soft toothbrush, toothpaste, baking soda, warm water in a glass, dental floss, and a bowl.

2. Bring the person to an upright position.

3. If possible, allow the person to clean his own teeth. This should be done twice daily and after meals.

4. Be sure the person can spit out water before allowing him to sip it. Use a water glass for rinsing.

5. If necessary, ask the person to open his mouth and gently brush the front and back teeth up and down.

6. Rinse well by having him sip water and spit into a bowl.

Oral Care for Someone Who Is Terminally Ill

If your doctor or nurse approves, use hydrogen peroxide diluted with mouthwash or a glycerin/water solution for mouth rinsing. Plain water is best for those who are very sensitive. Your pharmacist can give advice on a gentle mouthwash.

1. Gather supplies—latex gloves, toothettes (foam mouth-swabs), mouthwash, warm water in a glass, and a bowl.

2. Cleanse the mouth (roof, tongue, lips, and cheeks) with the disposable toothbrush.

3. Swab the mouth with a toothette dipped in water and repeat until the foam is gone.

4. If the lips are dry, apply a light coat of Vaseline.

Denture Cleaning

1. Remove the dentures from the mouth.

2. Run them under water and soak them in cleaner in a denture cup.

3. Rinse the person's mouth with water or mouthwash.

4. Stimulate the gums with a very soft toothbrush.

5. Return the dentures to the person's mouth.

NOTE Even a person with dentures should regularly visit the dentist to check the soft tissues of the mouth.

Foot Care

For the comfort and good health of the person in your care:

- Provide properly fitting low-heeled shoes with Velcro® or elastic closures and non-slip soles. Avoid shoes with heavy soles, running shoes with rubber tips over the toes, and shoes with thick cushioning which can make an older person fall.

- Provide cotton socks rather than acrylic.

- Trim the person's nails only after a bath when they have softened.

- Use a disposable sponge-tipped tooth brush to clean or dry between the toes.

- Check feet daily for bumps, cuts, and red spots.

Call the doctor or your health care provider if a sore develops on the foot. The diabetic must have special foot care to prevent infections from developing, because these may result in the amputation of a foot.

NOTE Foot pain can cause a person to lean back on his or her heels and increase the chance of a fall, so keep toenails trimmed and feet healthy.

Common Leg and Foot Problems and Solutions

Problem	Solution
Foot Strain	Visit a chiropodist.
Calluses	Rub lanolin or lotion on the area; do not cut hard skin.
Cramps	Relieve by movement and massage.
Hammer Toes and Bunions	Wedge a pad between the big toe and the second toe to straighten them; cut holes in the shoe to relieve rubbing.
Leg Ulcers (openings in the skin)	Follow the doctor's instructions. Exercise to keep the foot and ankle mobile.
Swollen Legs	Follow the doctor's instructions for treatment of the underlying cause.
Varicose Veins	Elevate the legs twice a day for 30 minutes. Before lowering the legs, apply an elastic bandage or stocking.

Dressing

Dressing a person with disabilities can be made easier by establishing a routine. Before you begin, lay the clothes out in the order they will be put on.

- Dress the person while she is sitting.

- Use adaptive equipment like a button hook and shoe horn. (📖 See *Equipment and Supplies*, page 128.)

- Avoid clothes with busy patterns. They may make it more difficult for the person to find buttons and zippers.

- Use loose clothes that are easy to put on and have elastic waistbands, Velcro® fasteners, and front openings.

- Use bras with front closures.

- Use tube socks.

- Dress the weak side first.

- For a bedridden person, use a gown with a back closure (for ease of opening when using a bedpan or urinal).

 NOTE For a bedridden person, be sure to eliminate all wrinkles in the clothes and bedding by smoothing out the fabric so as to prevent pressure sores from developing.

Dressing Someone With **Alzheimer's**

- If the person likes the same clothes, buy duplicates.

- Store all like clothes together.

- Simplify the person's wardrobe.

- Lay out clothing in the order that it is to be put on.

- Alter favorite clothing by replacing buttons with Velcro® closures.

- Use socks rather than pantyhose.

- Use nightgowns with overlapping back closures.

- Avoid clothes that have to be put on over the head.

Bed Making

Making a bed with someone in it can be relatively easy if you follow these steps:

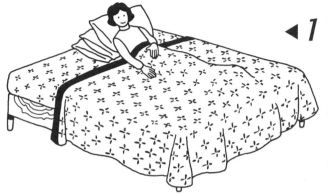

◄ **1**
- Look at the bed as having two parts—the side a person is lying on and the side you are making.

- If you have a hospital bed, raise the height of the bed.

- Lower the head and foot of the bed to make it flat.

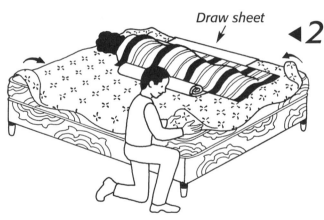

Draw sheet

◄ **2**
- Loosen the sheets on all sides.

- Remove the blankets and pillow, leaving only the bottom and top sheet.

- Cover the person with a bath blanket (a flannel sheet or large towel for modesty and warmth).

- Pull the top sheet out from under the bath blanket.

- Raise the bed rail on the side opposite you so the person cannot fall out of bed. If you don't have a hospital bed, be sure the bed is pushed against the wall.

- Roll the person over to the opposite side of the bed.

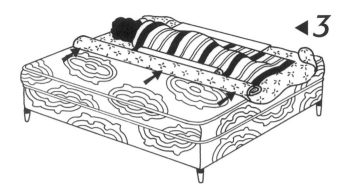

◄3
- Roll all the old bottom sheeting toward the person.

Clean sheet

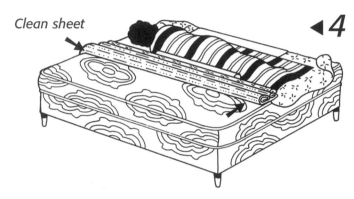

◄4
- Fold the clean sheet, along with other mattress covers, lengthwise.

- Place it on the bed with the middle fold running along the center of mattress right beside the person's body.

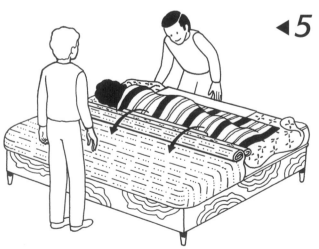

◄5
- Unfold the clean sheet and bring enough of it toward you to cover half of the bed.

- Gently lift the mattress and tuck the sheet in.

- Tuck the free edge of the draw sheet under the mattress on your side of the bed.

- Ask the person to roll over the linen in the middle of bed to the clean side.

OR

- Bend as close to the person's body as possible, place your hand and arm under the person's shoulders, and move the person and the bath blanket over the hump of linen in the center of the bed.

- If a hospital bed, raise the bed rail on your side and lock it into place.

- Go to the other side and remove all soiled linen. Tuck in all the linen and pull tight on the sheets to remove all wrinkles (which can rub and irritate the skin).

- Change the pillow case.

- Spread the top sheet over the person and bath blanket.

- Ask the person to hold the sheet while you pull the bath blanket away.

- Tuck the sheet under the mattress at the foot of the bed.

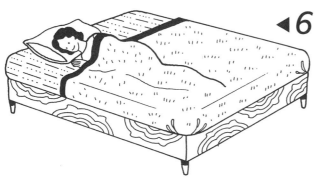

◀ 6

- Spread a blanket over the top. (The blanket should be high enough to cover the person's shoulders.)

- Fold the sheet down over the blanket.

- Adjust the person in bed so she is comfortable.

Toileting

Always wear latex gloves when helping with toileting. This prevents the spread of disease. Wash your hands before and after providing care.

Toileting in Bed

When a person is mobile, toileting in bed should not be encouraged.

Toileting in Bed for a Female or for Bowel Movements

1 •. Warm the bedpan with warm water then empty the water into the toilet.

•. Powder the bedpan with talcum powder to keep the skin from sticking to it.

•. Place a tissue or water in the pan to make cleaning easier. Or a light spray of vegetable oil in the bedpan will help the contents empty easily and completely.

• Raise the person's gown.

◀***2*** • Ask the person to raise her hips.

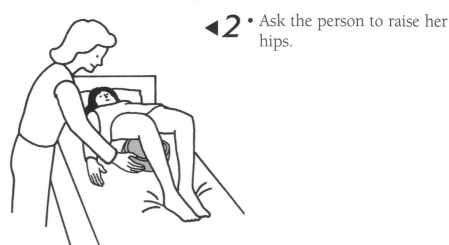

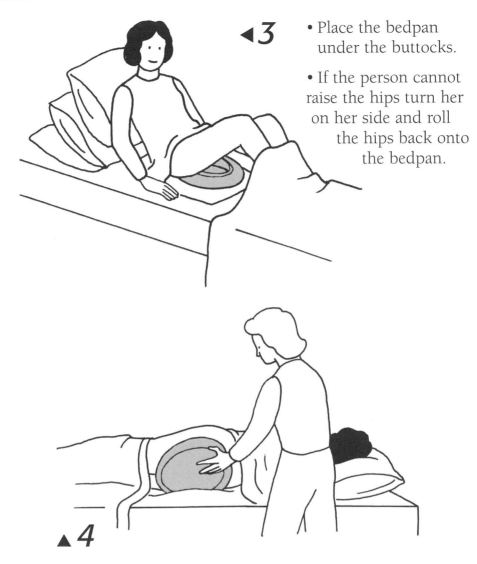

◄3

• Place the bedpan under the buttocks.

• If the person cannot raise the hips turn her on her side and roll the hips back onto the bedpan.

▲4

• If the person cannot do so, clean the anal area with bathroom tissue and then a wet tissue to keep the area clean.

• After the woman has urinated, pour a cup of warm water over her genitals and pat the area dry with a towel.

• Wash the person's hands.

• Remove and empty the bedpan.

• Be sure to wash your hands.

Using a Urinal

1. If the person can't do so himself, place the penis into the urinal as far as possible and hold it in.

2. When the person signals he is finished, remove and empty the urinal.

3. Wash his hands.

4. Wash your own hands.

Using a Commode

A portable commode is helpful for a person with limited mobility. The portable commode (with the pail removed) can be used over the toilet seat and as a shower seat.

Using a Portable Commode

1. Gather the portable commode, toilet tissue, a basin, a cup of water, a washcloth or paper towel, soap, and a towel.

2. Wash your hands.

3. Help the person onto the commode.

4. Offer toilet tissue.

5. Pour a cup of warm water on female genitalia.

6. Pat the area dry with a paper towel.

7. Offer a washcloth so the person can wash her hands.

8. Remove the pail from under the seat, empty it, rinse it with clear water, and empty the water into the toilet.

9. Wash your hands.

TOILET SAFETY
Use adhesive-backed Velcro® attached to the back of the toilet or commode seat to keep the lid from falling.

Using the Bathroom Toilet

If you find the mobile person is missing the toilet, a toilet seat in a contrasting color from the floor may help him see the toilet. If he is failing to cleanse the anal area, or failing to wash his hands, encourage these functions as tactfully as you can to prevent the spread of infections.

Catheters

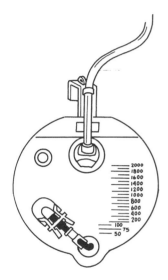

A urinary catheter is inserted by a nurse through the urethra into the bladder. It is made from plastic or rubber and drains urine from the body.

A foley catheter stays in the bladder and drains into a bag attached to a person's leg, the bed, or a chair. When caring for someone with an indwelling catheter, watch for these things:

1. Be sure the tube stays straight and drains properly. Check for kinks in the tubing.

2. Be sure the level of urine in the bag increases.

3. Be sure the drainage bag is always lower than the bladder.

4. Use tape or straps when securing a catheter to someone's inner thigh.

5. An erection in males is a common reaction to the catheter.

6. Notify the doctor if blood or sediment appears in the tubing or bag.

> **NOTE** A foley catheter greatly increases the risk of infection. It is chosen as a last resort in the management of incontinence.

Care of the Person Who Has a Catheter

1. Wash your hands.

2. Put on gloves.

3. Position the person on her back.

4. Take care not to pull on the catheter.

5. While holding the catheter, wash the area around it with a washcloth.

6. To avoid infection, wipe toward the anus, not back and forth.

NOTE To prevent foul odors from developing due to the growth of bacteria in the urine drainage bag, put a few drops of hydrogen peroxide in the bag when it is emptied.

Changing a Catheter from Straight Drainage to Leg Bag

1. Gather supplies—latex gloves, a bed protector, alcohol wipes, and a leg bag with straps.

2. Expose the end of the catheter and draining tubing; put a towel or other bed protector under this area.

3. Disconnect the drainage tubing from the catheter.

4. Wipe the attachment tube of the leg bag with an alcohol swab and insert it into the catheter.

5. Place the cap attached to the urinary drainage bag over the end of the tubing to keep it clean and prevent urine from leaking out

6. Secure the tubing to the person's leg.

Condom Catheter

A condom catheter may be prescribed by the doctor for a male if infections with the indwelling catheter become a chronic problem. The catheter fits over the penis like a condom. Unfortunately, leakage is often a problem with this type of aid.

Incontinence

Incontinence—the involuntary leakage of urine or an involuntary bowel movement—is a symptom, not a disease, and should never be treated as a normal consequence of aging. It can be caused by stroke, Multiple Sclerosis, infection, vaginitis, injury to the pelvic region, diseases involving brain cells or nerves to the bladder, or willful incontinence due to laziness and confusion. Treatments include bladder training, exercises to strengthen the pelvic floor (Kegel exercises), biofeedback, surgery, electrical muscle conditioner, urinary catheter, prosthetic devices, or external collection devices. Talk to the doctor about possible treatments for the person in your care.

To Manage Incontinence:

- Avoid alcohol, coffee, spicy foods, and citrus foods, which irritate the bladder and can cause prompt urination.

- Give fluids at regular intervals to dilute the urine. This decreases the irritation of the bladder

- Be sure the person in your care voids at regular intervals (ideally every 2 hours). Use an alarm clock to keep track of the time.

- Provide clothing that can be easily removed.

- Keep a bedpan or a portable commode in or near the bed.

- Provide absorbent products (adult diapers) to be worn under clothes.

- Stroke or tap the lower abdomen to cause voiding.

- Keep the skin dry and clean, because urine on the skin can cause pressure sores and infection.

- Your patience and understanding will foster self-confidence and respect.

A precise diagnosis for incontinence must be made in order to develop an effective treatment plan. If the primary care doctor does not adequately address the problem, consult an experienced urologist.

Urinary Tract Infection

Urinary tract infection may be present if the person has:

- blood in the urine

- a burning feeling when voiding

- cloudy urine with sediment

- cramping in the lower abdomen or side

- fever and chills

- foul-smelling urine

- a frequent, intense urge to void or frequent voiding

- pain in the lower back

Contact the doctor if symptoms persist.

Optimal Bowel Function

Maintaining good bowel function can be challenging, especially in elderly or bedridden individuals who get little exercise. For optimal bowel function:

- Establish a set time for bowel movements every day or every other day.

- Avoid foods high in fat and sugar.

- Serve fruits, vegetables, and bran.

- Be sure the person in your care drinks 2 quarts (eight glasses) of water daily (or an amount directed by the doctor).

- Provide opportunities for daily exercise.

- Use a stool softener or bulk agent if the stools are too hard. When using a bulk laxative, be sure that 6 to 8 glasses of water are taken per day. Otherwise there is a chance of severe constipation.

- Use glycerin suppositories as needed to help lubricate the bowels for ease of elimination.

- Clear the lower bowel with a 6 oz. warm water enema or a purchased enema. (Ask the pharmacist for advice.)

- Massage the abdomen in a clockwise direction. This can stimulate a bowel movement.

Diarrhea

Diarrhea (loose, watery stools) occurs when the intestines push stool along before water in them can be reabsorbed by the body. This condition can be caused by viral stomach flu, antibiotics, or stress anxiety.

To counteract diarrhea, consider two types of anti-diarrheals:

- those that thicken the stool

- those that slow intestinal spasms

Ask the pharmacist for advice.

Precautions:

- Do not use for the first 6 hours after diarrhea begins.

- Do not use if a fever is present.

- Stop taking as soon as the stool thickens.

- Encourage fluids to prevent dehydration.

Hemorrhoids

Hemorrhoids involve swelling and inflammation of veins around the anus. When they occur there is tenderness, pain, and bleeding. To treat hemorrhoids, you should:

- Be sure to keep anal area clean with pre-moistened tissues.

- Apply zinc oxide or petroleum jelly to the area.

- Relieve itching by using cold compresses on the anus for 10 minutes several times a day.

- Ask the doctor about suppositories.

Call the Doctor if the Following Symptoms Are Found in the Anus or Rectum:

- Blood from the hemorrhoids is dark red or brown and heavy.

- Bleeding continues for more than one week.

- Bleeding seems to occur for no reason.

Control of Infection in the Home

Bacteria, viruses, and fungi are micro-organisms that destroy human tissue by feeding on it and giving off waste products called toxins. The increase in infectious diseases and a growing resistance to antibiotics are renewing the need for common health practices such as frequent hand washing.

To minimize the chance of infection:
- Always work from the cleanest to the dirtiest area.
- Always wash your hands before and after contact with the person in your care and with other people.
- Always wear latex gloves when giving personal care.
- Always wash hands well when returning from a trip outside the house.
- Always wash your hands after using the toilet.

Cleaning Techniques

The following techniques will help cut the chance of infection in the home.

Caregiver Handwashing

- Handwashing is the single most effective way to prevent the transfer of infection or germs.

- Use antibacterial, bottle-dispensed soap.

- If the person in your care has an infection, use antimicrobial soap.

- Rub your hands for at least 30 seconds to produce lots of lather. Do this away from running water so the lather is not washed away.

- Use a nail brush on your nails; keep nails trimmed.

- Wash front and back of hands, between fingers and at least 2 inches up your wrists.

- Repeat the process.

- Dry your hands on a clean towel or a paper towel.

Precautions for Anyone Who Propels His or Her Own Wheelchair

- Wear leather gloves.

- Wash your hands frequently.

- For frequent in-between washings, use pre-packaged cleansing towelettes.

Soiled Laundry Handling

- Do not carry soiled linen close to your body.

- Never never shake dirty items or put soiled linens on the floor because they can contaminate the floor and germs will be spread throughout the house on the soles of shoes.

- Store infected soiled linen in a leak-proof plastic bag and tie it shut.

- Bag soiled laundry in the same place where it is used.

- Wash soiled linen separately from other clothes.

- Fill the machine with hot water, add bleach (no more than 1/4 cup) and detergent, rinse twice, then dry.

- Clean the washer by running it through a cycle with one cup bleach or other disinfectant.

- Use rubber gloves when handling soiled laundry.

- Wash your hands.

 If urine is highly concentrated because of bladder infection or dehydration, do not use bleach. The concentration of ammonia in the urine and bleach can cause toxic fumes.

Sterilization
If you are sharing equipment with other members of the family, sterilization will cut down on infection. If the person in your care is the only one using the equipment, wiping it with a cotton ball soaked in alcohol is adequate.

Wet Heat Sterilization

1. Fill a large pot with water.

2. If sterilizing glass pieces, put a cloth in the bottom of the pot.

3. Put items to be sterilized in the pot. These might include syringes, nail trimmers, and scissors for bandages.

4. Cover the pot and bring the water to a boil.

5. Boil undisturbed and covered for 20 minutes.

6. Leave the items in the pot until ready to use.

 NOTE Cloth can be sterilized by a hot iron held on it for a few seconds. Never use the microwave oven to disinfect any non-food items. They can catch fire or explode.

Disposal of Body Fluids

- Wear gloves (recommended for handling all body fluids).

- Flush liquid and solid waste down the toilet.

- Place used dressings and disposable pads in a sturdy plastic bag, tie securely, and place in a sealed receptacle for collection by the garbage hauler.

Prevention of Odors Caused by Bacteria

Bacteria needs moisture, warm body temperature, oxygen, darkness, and nourishment to grow. Some strong odors may be eliminated by:

- Sprinkling baking soda on the wound dressing.

- Leaving a full or partially full can of finely ground coffee open under the bed.

- Pouring a few drops of mouthwash in commodes and bedpans.

- Placing mouthwash-saturated cotton balls in the room.

- Spraying a fine mist of a solution of white distilled vinegar mixed with a few drops of eucalyptus or peppermint essential oil.

- Saturating cotton balls with vanilla extract and placing them in containers that retain strong odors.

- Using electrical and mechanical devices for removing odor.

- Buying natural organic commercial sprays.

Skin Care and Prevention of Pressure Sores

Pressure sores (also called decubiti or bed sores) are blisters or breaks in the skin caused when the body's weight presses blood out of a certain area. The most likely candidates for pressure sores are people who are low weight, overweight, malnourished, diabetic, dehydrated, or whose bodies retain fluids. The best treatment of pressure sores is prevention. How much time they take to heal depends on how advanced the condition is.

Facts

- The most common areas for sores are the bony areas—tail bone, hips, heels, and elbows.

- Sores can appear when the skin rubs repeatedly on a sheet.

- The skin breakdown starts from inside, works up to the surface, and can occur in just 15 minutes.

- Damage can range from a change in color in unbroken skin to deep wounds down to the muscle or bone.

- In light-skinned people, in the first stage, a sore may change skin color to a dark purple or red area that does not become pale under fingertip pressure. In dark-skinned people, this area may become darker than normal.

- The affected area may feel warmer than surrounding skin.

- Untreated pressure sores can lead to hospitalization and can require skin grafts.

Prevention

- Check the skin daily. (Bath time is the ideal time to do this without causing a person discomfort.)

- Provide a well-balanced diet, with adequate vitamin C, zinc, and protein.

- Keep the skin dry and clean (urine left on the skin can cause sores and infection).

- Keep clothing loose.

- If splints or braces are used, make sure they are adjusted properly.

- Massage the body with light pressure using equal parts surgical spirit and glycerin. (Ask a nurse or a pharmacist for advice.)

- Turn a bedridden person at least every 2 hours, alternating positions. Keep wrinkles out of sheets.

- Lightly tape foam to bony sections of the body using paper tape, which will not hurt the skin when peeled off.

- Use flannel or 100% cotton sheets to absorb moisture.

- Provide an egg crate or sheepskin mattress pad for added comfort.

- Rent an electrically operated ripple bed (with sections that inflate alternately).

- Avoid using a plastic sheet or a Chux if they cause sweating.

- When the person is sitting, encourage changing the body position every 15 minutes.

- Use foam pads on chair seats to cushion the buttocks.

- Change the type of chair the person sits in; occasionally try an open-back garden chair.

- Provide as much exercise as possible.

WOUND PREVENTION

If a person has a tendency to scratch or pick at a spot, have him wear cotton gloves. (Make sure the hands are clean and dry before putting the gloves on.)

When Turning Someone in Bed to Minimize Sores:

1. Explain to the person what you are doing.

2. If possible, raise the bed to its highest position.

3. Lower the head of the bed to a flat position.

4. Loosen the draw sheet at the far side.

5. Stand in proper alignment as close to the person as possible.

6. Roll the far side of the draw sheet toward you and up close to the person's side.

7. Prop a pillow against his back.

8. Flex his knees slightly.

9. Place one pillow between the knees and another between the feet.

10. Check any catheter tubing.

Treatment

If, in your daily observations of the skin, you see pressure sores, you must alert the nurse or the doctor. General guidelines for treatment of these sores are as follows:

Where Pressure Sores Can Appear

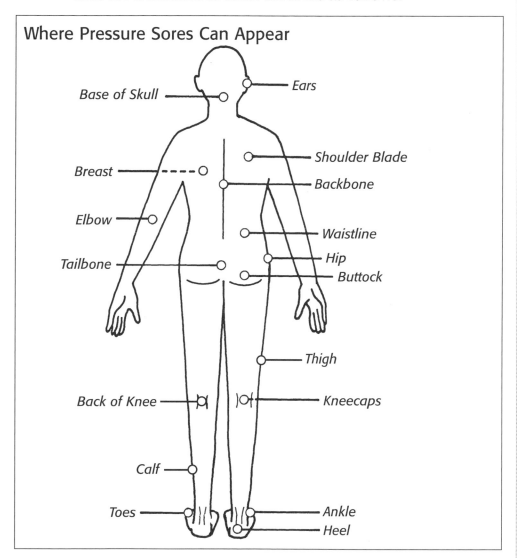

- To reduce the chance of infection, provide all care while wearing gloves.

- Take constant pressure off sores by changing positions often and by using pillows or a foam pad to support the body with at least one inch of padding.

191

- Do not position the person on his bony parts.

- Do not let the person lie on pressure sores.

- In bed, change positions at least every two hours.

- Follow the doctor's or nurse's treatment plan in applying medication to sores and bandaging the areas to protect them while they heal.

Eating

Mealtimes are important times for people who are elderly or ill because they provide a welcome diversion in the day. If it is not too distracting for the person in your care, have her eat with the family. Expect and ignore spills and less-than-perfect manners. It is important that mealtimes are enjoyable so that eating is encouraged.

If a person eats alone or has disabilities, she often suffers needlessly from malnutrition. Look for these free or low-cost solutions:

Community meals—local meal programs sponsored by the federal government and open to anyone over 59 and the person's spouse (call your local Area Agency on Aging or Department of Welfare and Human Resources)

Meals-on-Wheels—hot meals delivered to the home (call the Visiting Nurse Association)

Food Stamps—help based on income that can stretch food dollars (call Department of Welfare and Human Resources or the Area Agency on Aging)

For best results at meal times:

- Allow 30–45 minutes for eating.

- Avoid cluttered meal presentation.

- Make sure all items are ready to eat and within reach.

- Provide a consistent, comfortable table/chair or other eating arrangement.

- Supply easy-to-hold eating utensils. To avoid cuts, throw out all chipped cups and plates.

- Minimize excess noise such as television and radio.

- If vision is poor, be consistent with where food is placed on the plate.

Feeding Someone in Bed

1. Prop the head with pillows.

2. Provide an over-the-bed table.

3. Do not rush feeding, but maintain a steady pace.

4. Cut the food into bite-size portions.

5. Explain what food is served.

6. Fill cups only half full.

7. Let the person hold the cup if she wants to. (A terry cloth tennis wrist band slipped over the cup may make it easier to hold.)

8. Use available eating aids. (See *Equipment and Supplies,* page 127.)

9. Keep a moistened hand towel to gently wipe the person's mouth and hands. Chains used for eyeglasses can hold a napkin in place.

FEEDING IN BED

An adjustable ironing board may be used as an over-the-bed table for activities or eating.

Feeding the Helpless Person or the Person With *Alzheimer's*

1. Name the food being offered.

2. If the person plays with food, limit the choices being offered. (Playing with food occurs because a person is confused and unable to make choices.)

3. Check the temperature of the food often.

4. Be gentle with forks and spoons. (A rubber-tipped baby spoon may be helpful.)

5. Feed at a steady pace, alternating food and drink.

6. Remove a spoon from the person's mouth very slowly. If the person clenches the spoon, let go of it and wait for the jaw to relax.

7. Give simple instructions such as "open your mouth," "move your tongue," "now swallow."

8. If the person spits food out, try feeding later.

9. If the person refuses food, provide a drink and return in 10 minutes with the food tray.

10. Between meals, provide a nourishing snack, such as stewed fruit, tapioca pudding, or finger foods.

Boosting Food Intake When the Appetite Is Poor

- Offer more food at the time of day when the person is most hungry.

- To heighten the appeal of food for those with decreased taste and smell, provide strong flavors.

- Use milk or cream instead of water in soups and cooked cereal.

- Add fat through butter or margarine on foods.

- Add nonfat dry milk powder to foods like yogurt, mashed potatoes, gravy, and sauces.

- Encourage the person to eat with his fingers, if that is the only way to get him to eat.

- Offer supplemental milk or fruit shakes.

- Offer baby foods of one type (avoid combination dinners and puddings).

(See *Diet and Nutrition*, page 240.)

> **NOTE** If the person in your care needs to swallow three or four times with each bite of food; coughs before, during, or after swallowing; pockets food in his mouth; or senses something caught or sticking in the back of his throat, he may have a condition called dysphagia. Difficulty swallowing must be evaluated to determine if it is a symptom of a treatable condition and to help the caregiver learn proper feeding techniques.

Eating Problems and Solutions

Drooling—Use a straw if possible; help close the mouth with your hand. (However, sometimes use of straws can cause choking if liquid touches the back of the mouth too quickly.)

Spitting out food—Ask the doctor if the cause is moodiness or disease.

Excessive repetition in swallowing/chewing—Coach the person to alternate hot and cold bites.

Difficulty chewing—Use denture adhesive and change the diet to soft foods.

Difficulty swallowing—Put foods through a blender or food mill; avoid thin liquids and instead serve thick liquids such as milk shakes.

Eating with the fingers—Show the person how to use utensils.

Poor scooping—Use bowls instead of plates.

Difficulty cutting food—Use a small pizza cutter or rolling knife.

Trouble moving food to the back of the mouth—Change the food's consistency and demonstrate how to direct the food to the center of the mouth.

Excessively dry or wet mouth—Ask the doctor or the pharmacist if this is a side effect of medications.

A tendency to be easily distracted—Pull down the shades and remove the distractions.

 Difficulty swallowing can cause food or liquids to be taken into the lungs, which can lead to pneumonia. Reduce the chance of food entering the lungs by keeping the person in your care upright for at least 30 minutes after a meal.

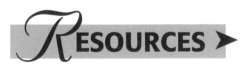 **ESOURCES** ➤

American Association of Oral and Maxillofacial Surgeons
www.aaoms.org
Provides self-examination and oral cancer patient information on the Web site.

National Association for Continence (NAFC)
P.O. Box 8310
Spartanburg, SC 29305-8310
(864) 579-7900
Fax (864) 579-7902
(800) 252-3337
www.nafc.org
NAFC is a leading source of education and support to the public about the diagnosis, treatments and management alternatives for incontinence.

If you don't have home access to the Internet, ask your local library to help you locate any Web site.

Therapies

Therapies

The following instructions are provided for your general knowledge. They do NOT substitute for training with professional therapists.

Physical Therapy

Physical therapy is part of the process of relearning how to function after an injury, illness, or period of inactivity. If muscles are not used, they shorten and tighten, making joint motion painful.

What a Physical Therapist Does

A physical therapist treats a patient to relieve pain, develop and restore muscle function, and maintain maximum performance using physical means such as active and passive exercise, massage, heat, water, and electricity. Broadly speaking, a physical therapist—

- establishes goals of treatment with patient and family

- shows how to use special equipment

- instructs in routine daily functions

- teaches safe ways to move

- sets up and teaches an exercise program

NOTE The American Physical Therapy Association, often located in the state capital, can provide a list of licensed therapists.

What a Physical Therapist Determines

Depending on a person's physical condition, a therapist may work on Range-of-Motion exercises, correct body positions when resting, devices to help stroke patients, and other simple ways to improve daily functions.

A physical therapist checks things that can affect a person's daily activities—

- his attitude toward his situation

- how well he can move his muscles and joints (Range of Motion)

- his ability to see, smell, hear, and feel

- what he can do on his own and what he needs to learn

- his equipment needs, now and later

- what can be improved in the home to make moving around safer and more comfortable

- who can and will help to give support

Range-of-Motion (ROM) Exercises

The purpose of Range-of-Motion exercises is to relieve pain, maintain normal body alignment, help prevent skin swelling and breakdown, and promote bone formation. A ROM exercise program should be started before deformities develop. When you are asked to help with exercises at home:

- Take each movement only as far as the joint will go into a comfortable stretch. (Mild discomfort is okay, but it should go away quickly.)

- Communicate what you are doing.

- Use the flats of both hands, not the fingertips, to hold a body part.

Joints Used in ROM

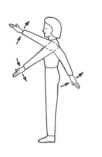

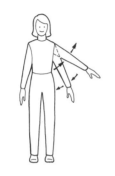

▲ shoulder

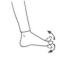

▲ feet, ankle, toe

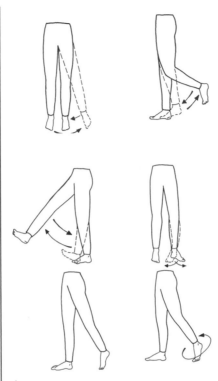

▲ hip

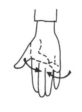

▲ hands

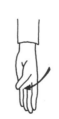

▲ wrists

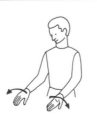

▲ elbows

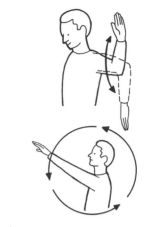

▲ shoulders

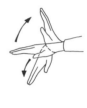

▲ finger/thumb

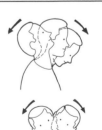

▲ neck

- Do each exercise 3–5 times.

- Use slow steady movements to help relax muscles and increase joint range.

- If joints are swollen and painful, exercise very gently.

Proper Positions to Use When Resting:

- flat on the back or no more than 30° elevated

- prone on the stomach
  (for up to 20–30 minutes only—not for sleeping)

- one-quarter left or right turn onto the back

- three-quarters right or left turn onto the stomach

- aided by special positioning devices (for example, splints for leg, foot, hand, or back support)

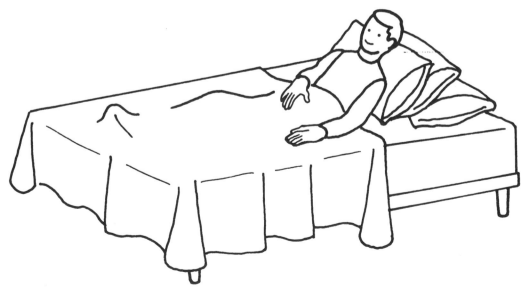

▲ *When resting keep head elevated no more than 30 degrees.*

Positioning Devices for Stroke Patients

Arm Trough—attaches to the arm of a wheelchair; provides support and positioning of the arm

Finger Spreader—keeps the hand in a relaxed position with the fingers spread

Lap Board—lies across both arms of a wheelchair; provides support and positioning

Resting Hand Splint—slowly relaxes muscles; keeps the hand in an open position with the thumb away from the palm

Shoulder Girdle Sling—holds the shoulder joint in a normal position

Sling—supports a flaccid arm (rarely used now)

Occupational Therapy

Occupational therapy is the health and rehabilitation profession designed to help people regain and build skills that are important for gaining functional independence. The occupational therapist will help the doctor evaluate levels of function.

The occupational therapist will:

- evaluate a person's strength, range of motion, endurance, and dexterity needed to do everyday tasks that were done easily before an illness or injury happened

- design a program of activities and functional solutions that assure maximum independence

- provide training to relearn everyday activities of daily living like eating, grooming, dressing, toileting, bathing, and leisure activities

- evaluate the need for special equipment—wheelchairs, feeding devices, transfer equipment, hand and skin devices

Speech Therapy

Speech therapy is the treatment of disorders of communication, including speaking, hearing, writing, reading, and communication required for the activities of daily living. Speech therapists also teach people to swallow foods and liquids safely.

A speech therapist or speech pathologist works to:

- strengthen weakened oral muscles through specific exercises

- teach techniques for basic communication

- teach a patient and family how to manage a communication or swallowing disorder

Specialized Therapies

Many types of therapy exist to help with special needs, both in the hospital and at home. They include:

Antibiotic Therapy—antibiotics infused into a vein to treat lingering infections

Chemotherapy—anti-cancer medication given through a lightweight infusion pump

Dialysis—machines to clean the blood in the case of kidney failure

Enteral Nutrition Therapy—liquid nutrition pumped through a thin feeding tube from the nose into the stomach or surgically placed into the small intestine by way of the abdomen

Enterostomal Therapy—training in the care of hard-to-heal sores, wounds and ostomy (an artificial opening in the abdomen for the removal of urine and stool)

Infusion Therapy—fluids for nutrition, antibiotics, or chemotherapy given intravenously

Respiratory Therapy—oxygen systems that help with breathing problems and keep lung function at its highest level

Total Parenteral Nutrition (TPN)—infusion of nutrients through a vein for one who cannot eat

Massage Therapy

Massage therapy is an aid to good health because it relaxes muscles, stimulates circulation, and releases stress. You can learn to give a simple massage; however, massage for cancer, HIV or AIDS-afflicted persons should be done only by a professional. Also, do not massage broken skin.

When you give a massage, use only natural oils (olive or almond)—never mineral oils or petroleum-based products like Vaseline.

Back Massage

- Wash your hands with warm water.

- Use warm massage oil or baby powder.

- Expose the back and buttocks.

- Apply oil to the entire back from shoulders to buttocks with long firm strokes.

- Use gentle circular motions on each area.

- Dry the back.

Hand Massage

- Wash your hands with warm water.

- Apply warm massage oil or lotion.

- Use short or medium strokes from wrist to fingertips.

- Gently squeeze all sides of the fingers from base to tip. Use this "milking" motion on the entire hand.

- Lay the person's hand on yours and gently draw your top hand toward you several times.

- Do not massage swollen or reddened portions of the hand.

 TREATING INFLAMMATION
If inflammation in the finger joints occurs, apply ice for the first 24 hours and provide an anti-inflammatory pain reliever, unless the person's condition does not allow it.

Horticultural Therapy

Gardening is one of the oldest healing arts. Horticultural therapy uses plants and gardening activities to help treat or strengthen an elderly person or a person with special needs. The goal is to improve mental and physical health and the person's spirits.

Advantages of Horticultural Therapy

- exercises eyes and body

- establishes leisure time activities to fill time left when other activities can no longer be pursued

- promotes interest and enthusiasm for the future

- provides topics of conversation

- motivates a person to walk and bend

- improves confidence

- provides a feeling of usefulness

- gives opportunities to daydream

- makes it possible to grow useful house plants or vegetables

- allows a person to be in the sunshine and (sometimes) hear soothing sounds of running water or birds

▶ *Gardening can be enjoyed by anyone.*

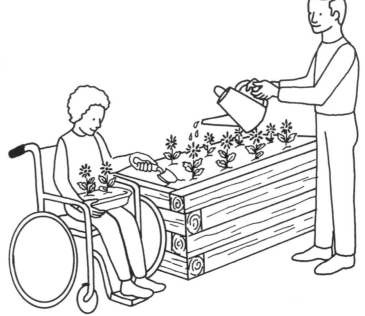

To Make Gardening Easier

Make sure that proper body mechanics are used. Avoid twisting the body, face in the direction of the work being done, and lift using the strength of the torso and legs. A leather weightlifter's belt can help provide back support.

- Use proper equipment—tools that are right for the person's height and strength.

- Avoid sunburn, chemicals, and hazardous plants.

- Use raised beds to minimize stooping or bending.

- Use perennials that do not have to be reseeded each year.

- Use seed tape or mechanical seed clickers to reduce the need to hold tiny seeds.

- Ensure that gardening walkways are 3 feet wide and have non-slip surfaces.

- For arthritis sufferers, provide gloves that are large enough to insert foam. The foam eases pain.

- Use tools with cushioned grips.

- Provide foam pads for kneeling or a small stool for sitting.

- To help prevent kneecap injury, avoid a squatting position. Have the person in your care sit on the ground and move backwards.

- Provide a timer as a reminder to mark 20 minutes when a body position should be changed to avoid repetitive motions.

 If the person in your care is in the garden alone, provide a whistle on a cord worn around the neck so he or she can call for help.

Aromatherapy

Aromatherapy is a branch of herbal medicine that uses the essential oils of various plants for medicinal purposes. Essential oils act to energize or pacify, help digestion, and remove toxins from the body.

Ways to Use Essential Oils

- with a diffuser—for those with some respiratory conditions

- through external application—in baths or massages (2 or 3 drops with almond or olive oil)

- in floral waters—sprayed on skin too sensitive to touch

Common Conditions to Treat with Essential Oils

- For insomnia, a room perfumed with lavender or rose in a diffuser is an effective treatment.

- For low energy, use geranium and peppermint.

- For relaxation, try cinnamon and chamomile diffused or rubbed on the wrists and temples.

- For positive associations for an elderly person, try the aroma of ginger, cloves, and allspice.

- To cleanse the respiratory system, use eucalyptus in a diffuser.

Essential oils can be expensive but because they are only used in drops, they last. Buy essential oils from a supplier or a health food store that specializes in them. Starter kits with the most widely used selections are available. Never drink essential oils or use them directly on the skin.

 People with medical conditions should consult their health professional before using essential oils.

Pet Therapy

A cat, bird, or dog can bring joy to people and provide companionship, relaxation, and an opportunity to exercise. They also provide a means to lessen the boredom and fear caused by loneliness.

- Before selecting a dog, check canine-assisted living programs in your area. Dogs that were rejected from the program may be ideal for a frail person.

- Choose a mature dog that is house trained; do not get a puppy.

- Have a dog or cat neutered to lessen the chance of roaming.

- Keep up all pet vaccinations.

- Never clean pet cages or feeding dishes in the kitchen sink.

 Be aware that animals carry bacteria and intestinal parasites, so the elderly and other individuals with weakened immune systems should not change the kitty litter box and should wash their hands frequently.

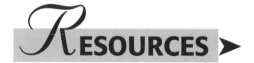

American Horticultural Therapy Association
909 York Street
Denver, CO 80206
(720) 865-3616
Fax (720) 865-3728
www.ahta.org
Support and education resource for people interested in horticultural therapy.

For more information on garden hints, call your local county office of the **Home Extension Service.**

NCM Consumer Products Division
(800) 235-7054
www.ncmedical.com
Sells garden tools that have special handles.

Charley's Greenhouse & Garden Supply
(800) 322-4707
www.charleysgreenhouse.com
Offers a variety of garden tools that are specially made for those with physical difficulties. Ask for "easy gardening" tools.

Gardenscape Tools
(888) 472-3266
www.gardenscapetools.com
Offers a variety of enabling tools.

Delta Society
289 Perimeter Road East
Renton, WA 98055-1329
(425) 226-7357
Fax (425) 235-1076
www.deltasociety.org
E-Mail: info@deltasociety.org
Provides information on the human-animal bond and information on how to obtain a service animal.

Contact your local **Humane Society** for information about pet therapy.

Special Challenges

Special Challenges

Communication

Communication is the ability to speak, understand speech, read, write, and gesture. Nonverbal messages are given through silence, body movements, or facial expression. Be aware that words can carry one message, the body another.

Loss of Speech in Stroke Patients

Loss of speech can happen due to damage to the brain or lack of oxygen. The person who experiences such a loss still has the same intelligence he or she had before the injury, though this fact may be hard to remember in light of dramatic changes in behavior.

- The communication problem may involve talking or understanding.

- The person may be able to say words at one time and then not at another, or may repeat the same word over and over.

- The person may unknowingly swear or laugh or cry frequently.

- Left-brain damage affects listening, speaking, reading, and writing.

- Right-brain damage affects non-linguistic skills such as assessing a situation and behaving appropriately, controlling facial expressions, and understanding tones of voice.

A speech therapist can suggest specific tasks to help the person communicate—for example,

- using pictures instead of words

- teaching specific exercises to strengthen the muscles of the face, lips, or tongue.

To communicate better with the stroke victim, try:

- getting the person's attention by lightly touching her arm before speaking

- speaking slowly and simply

- asking questions that require simple yes/no answers

- providing opportunities for the person to hear speech

- helping the person communicate frustrations

- pacing activities, because the person will tire easily

- not allowing the person to become bossy

Improving the Chance of Being Understood

When talking to a person with hearing loss follow these guidelines:

- Sit in the light so your lips and facial expressions can be seen.

- Make eye contact.

- Use simple sentences.

- Use body language (nodding, pointing) and lots of facial expression.

- Before starting a conversation, introduce what you are going to talk about ("Mom, lets talk about our vacation"). When you change the subject, say so ("Now lets talk about dinner").

- Speak louder without shouting. Shouting makes words more difficult to hear.

> **NOTE** If the person in your care has a buzzing in the ear called tinnitus, ask your health care professional about a tinnitus mask which drowns out the humming with "white noise." A loudly ticking clock or static of a radio can also create white noise.

Sexual Expression

A disability does not equate with loss of sexuality. The needs for intimacy and sharing do not change, although the ability to move in the usual manner may have changed. To improve your spouse's ability to exercise sexual expression, try to increase his or her self-esteem and downplay the role of "patient." Ask your health care professional about assistive devices and techniques for enhanced sexual activities.

AIDS and the Older Adult

AIDS is a disease caused by a virus called HIV. HIV attacks the body's immune system and when the immune system is damaged, it can no longer fight diseases. People with HIV seem healthy at first. As the disease progresses, they begin to get sick with infections. When this happens, they are diagnosed with AIDS.

Older people are at risk for AIDS. Symptoms include feeling confused, being tired, experiencing loss of appetite, and having swollen glands. If you suspect AIDS, find a doctor who knows about the latest research by calling your local medical school's department of infectious diseases for a list of experts.

Prevention of AIDS

In older people, sexual activity is the most common cause of HIV infection. The second most common cause is a blood transfusion received before 1985. Since 1985 blood banks have been testing all blood for HIV, so there is little danger of getting HIV from transfusions.

If you are caring for someone with HIV virus or AIDS or if you have the condition, follow some basic rules:

- Always use gloves when providing personal care or handling bodily fluids.

- Always use condoms with penetrative sex.

- Realize that HIV cannot be spread by being coughed or sneezed on by an infected person.

Depression

Aging is a healthy, normal process and not an illness. However, negative emotions and mental attitudes can result in disease. Personality changes with chronic illness can be dramatic, and people with worsening conditions can suffer personality changes that are as permanent as the disease. The most common mental health problems of the aged are depression, anxiety, dementia (e.g., Alzheimer's Disease), substance abuse, and paranoia. The suicide rate is higher for the elderly than for any other age group.

Old age is difficult because a person has to make adjustments due to loss of physical strength or health, retirement, death of a spouse, new living arrangements, and the need to accept and prepare for death.

NOTE Depression is often misdiagnosed as dementia or Alzheimer's, but there are differences. Also, several drugs and medical conditions can lead to memory loss. These problems can be reversed, so it is important to get a correct diagnosis for anyone suspected of having Alzheimer's or dementia.

Common Fears of a Person with a Long-Term Illness

- loss of self-image
- loss of control over life
- loss of independence and fear of abandonment
- fear of living alone and being lonely
- fear of death

You can help deal with these powerful emotions by:

- pointing out the person's strengths and focusing on small successes
- restoring areas of control to the person by giving as many choices as possible
- finding new ways for the person to adjust to limitations
- providing insight into sources of meaning in life
- changing your attitude about the person's disability
- recognizing that humor is healing and providing large doses of laughter to stimulate a positive attitude, providing humorous books, comics, cartoons, television, or movies
- allowing the person to cry at hearing news of a diagnosis
- allowing for the power of silence
- providing opportunities for peer support and friendship (which works exceptionally well with the elderly)

Seasonal Affective Disorder

Some depression can be brought on by the dark, gloomy days of winter. This type of depression may be treated by sitting in front of full-spectrum lights for one hour per day. However, be wary of gadgets that promise miraculous results.

Dealing with Boredom

Boredom is another problem for people who are ill, and fighting it can take all your creativity. Try—

- watching funny movies

- taking car or bus trips

- listening to music, especially from the person's youth

- taking up hobbies

- going to social events

- playing board games and card games

- attending public library discussion clubs and using large print or talking books

- joining activist organizations like the League of Women Voters and Gray Panthers

- spending time with others in similar difficulties—in religious groups, recreation centers, stroke clubs (contact the National Stroke Association), or the YMCA/YWCA

- being involved in volunteer service organizations such as the Retired & Senior Volunteer Program

- using a computer and accessing sites on the Internet (which helps prevent loneliness through interesting activity and provides the ability to communicate with family and friends through e-mail)

Continuing Education

Attending continuing education classes at local colleges or correspondence schools can provide education opportunities, even for shut-ins. There are opportunities for both academic and nonacademic classes (for example, boat building, ceramics and garden design).

To find the program that fits your needs:

- Check college programs in your area.

- Check organizations such as museums, botanical gardens and arts groups.

- Check Internet listings devoted to distance learning.

- Check PBS Adult Service Online, which offers college courses based on their documentaries.

- Check high school evening courses.

TUITION DISCOUNTS

Some states are encouraging older students to attend college by offering tuition discounts at public institutions.

The Internet and Computers

A TV set-top Internet box is a device that enables a person to use the TV to connect to the World Wide Web. With just 3 wires to connect—one to the electrical outlet, one to the TV, and one to the telephone line—the Internet box provides a low-cost, simple way for seniors to use the Internet or electronic mail to stay in touch with family and friends.

If you want more features and are able to spend a little more, consider a computer for the person in your care. A computer is ideal for the person who has difficulty writing, and it can make life simpler for anyone through these features—

- enabling a person to type instead of write letters

- providing easy duplication of letters by personalizing each letter for the recipient

- avoiding costly long distance telephone charges by communicating with friends and family using electronic mail (e-mail)

- enabling a person to shop via the computer

- tracking household and investments accounts

- paying bills by computer-printed checks instead of hand written ones

- having ones access to the Internet for information about a limitless array of subjects

Computer software is available that helps users who are visually impaired, deaf, or have other disabilities.

TECHNOLOGY

Check the local library for computers-for-seniors classes or for help locating any Web site.

Consumer Fraud and The Lure of Sweepstakes

Lonely elderly people are especially vulnerable to fraudulent telephone solicitations that offer the hope of winning a cash sweepstakes or that appeal to their sense of charity. Some—usually those who are widowed and isolated from their families—even become "addicted" to the attention of tele-marketers. These victims are often concerned that their savings will not cover all their living costs and see grand prizes as their only hope.

To help an elderly person who may become a victim of fraud, suggest that certain common-sense rules be followed when receiving calls from telephone solicitors:

- Be wary of a caller who is overly friendly and calls you by your first name.

- Be wary of a caller who insists that you act immediately.

- Be wary of any caller who asks you to send a check by Western Union or overnight delivery.

- Be wary of calls before 8:00 a.m., after 9:00 p.m., or during the weekend.

- Never buy anything by telephone unless *you* made the call.

- Never give out your credit card number unless *you* have made the call.

- Never give out your bank account, Social Security, Medicare, or Medicaid number over the telephone or to people you do not know.

- Never contribute to an organization over the telephone, even if you are familiar with the name. Ask the caller to send you a written request.

- If the caller says that phoning saves the charity postage costs, insist the solicitation is sent in writing.

- Be wary of free gifts requiring that you pay shipping charges—your credit card may billed for items you don't want.

- Beware of a request to prepay taxes on a prize. In legitimate awards the sweepstakes promoter will withhold taxes or report your winnings to the Internal Revenue Service.

- Be wary of securities, investment, or home repair offers that sound too good to be true. Ask for written confirmation of the service or investment opportunity. Consult with a friend or relative before making a decision.

- Do not take money from your bank account if a stranger asks you to—even if he says he is a bank employee and is testing a bank teller.

- Do not allow anyone to send a messenger to your home to pick up a payment.

- Do not fall prey to fraudulent solicitors. JUST HANG UP.

- Check offers by calling the National Consumer League's **National Fraud Information Center** at (800) 876-7060 or the local consumer protection office.

- If you continue to receive phone calls from the same company, call your local Better Business Bureau and the state Attorney General's office to report the name of the company.

(📖 See *Equipment and Supplies,* page 117.)

To be removed from national telemarketing telephone lists write the

Telephone Preference Center
Direct Marketing Association
P.O. Box 9014
Farmingdale, NY 11735-9008

To be removed from national mailing lists write the

Mail Preference Service
Direct Marketing Association
P.O. Box 9008
Farmingdale, NY 11735-9008

Include your full name and telephone number as well as any variations such as J. Brown, Mrs. James Brown, etc. Consider collecting the labels from all junk mail for a few months, taping them to a sheet of paper, mailing it to the service, and requesting that all the listed variations be removed. The service is updated quarterly so it will take a few months for your request to be processed.

To be taken off the Department of Motor Vehicles mailing list, contact your local DMV office.

NOTE To avoid the chance of theft or misplacement, have monthly pension or Social Security checks deposited directly to the bank account.

Pain Management

Pain is an individual experience that is tied to both physical and mental states. Even noise makes a person tense, which can contribute to pain. Fatigue, depression, and anxiety can make pain harder to tolerate. (Lying in bed does not lessen the pain, although it may appear that the person is comfortable and relaxed.)

Types of Pain

Pain falls into two categories:

Acute—short-term pain from illness or injury, which can be managed with prescribed narcotics and will subside when the injury heals

Chronic—pain that begins with an illness, is long-term (more than six months), and is controlled with medications, which may create other problems as the tolerance of those medications increases

Pain can be described as—

- sharp

- stabbing

- hot

- a dull ache

- constant or intermittent

- occurring in a specific location and unrelieved by changing position or by rest

- associated with numbness or extreme weakness

Pain Reduction Techniques

The most effective methods for relieving pain are pain medications (analgesics), sleep, immobilization, and distraction.

(Also, heat and cold increase or decrease circulation to the affected area, but should not be used without specific instructions from a doctor.)

To reduce pain, consider:

- distraction through TV, music, or reading aloud

- distraction from a medical procedure by massaging the person's hand

- reduction of stress and promotion of healing through relaxation, meditation, and prayer

 Although good nutrition will not relieve pain, it promotes healing by strengthening the body.

Pain can be controlled through the following techniques:

- **Acupuncture**—insertion of needles into designated points of the body

- **Acupressure**—pressure and massage at acupuncture points

- **Biofeedback**—the monitoring of reactions to conscious and subconscious thoughts by measuring changes in blood pressure, temperature, and body organs

- **Deep Breathing**—slow deep breaths taken through the nose and exhaled slowly through pursed lips (relieves pain by increasing oxygen to brain)

- **Drugs**—narcotics provide very strong relief but can be addicting if taken long term

- **Hypnosis**—an altered state of consciousness that replaces a focus on pain with attention to another idea

- **Meditation**—a technique for visualizing relief from pain

- **Placebo**—a "sugar" pill that fools the body into thinking it is taking a pain killer and signals pain relief

- **Psychic Healing**—a technique known as "laying on of hands" that, according to new scientific studies, actually can transfer healing energy to another person's body

- **Psychotic Transfer**—a technique that involves having two people go into a meditative state so they can "transfer" pain from one to the other

- **Surgery**—permanent severing of nerves to block pain (a step that requires careful consideration)

- **Topical Pain Relievers**—creams, rubs, or sprays applied to muscles or joints for pain relief in a specific area

- **Transcutaneous Nerve Stimulator (TNS)**—an electronic device placed over acupuncture points

 NOTE Sound sleep is often interrupted in older people because of chronic pain and other discomforts. Since a person does not require less sleep as he or she ages, expect more naps during the day.

Transportation and Travel

Transportation

There is a network of transportation services, public and private, that will pick up the disabled and the elderly at their homes. These services rely on vans and paid drivers and run on a schedule to specific locations. Free transportation is available from community volunteer organizations, although most public services charge on a sliding scale.

Many states ensure transportation to necessary medical care for Medicaid recipients. Check with your local Medicaid office to see if you qualify.

Community transportation services are provided by:

- home health care agencies
- public health departments
- religious organizations
- civic clubs
- the local American Red Cross
- the Area Agency on Aging
- local public transportation companies

Travel

Some group tours and cruise lines cater to the elderly or disabled traveler. Before traveling long distances with a person who has a chronic condition, however, consult the person's doctor.

TRAVEL PLANNING

If you, as the primary caregiver, are traveling for an extended period, consider investing in a long-distance pager with a toll-free pager number so you can be reached in case of emergency.

Travel Emergencies

In the event of an emergency abroad, contact American Citizen Services (ACS) in the foreign offices of American consulates and embassies.

American Citizens Services will assist with:

- lists of doctors, dentists, hospitals, and clinics

- informing the family if an American becomes ill or injured while traveling

---

Checklist **Travel for the Person with a Chronic Condition**

✓ Let the person's primary care doctor know of your travel plans.

✓ Take more of the person's medications than needed, along with a list of names and dosages.

✓ Check with the doctor to see if an immunization against Hepatitis A is recommended if traveling to high-risk areas.

✓ Take a list of all medical conditions.

✓ Use a Medic-Alert identification bracelet for the person in care.

✓ Take a copy of his EKG.

✓ Read his insurance policy before taking the trip to see how "emergency" is defined.

✓ If medical care is needed during the trip, get copies of all bills to support claims for reimbursement.

✓ Check into reciprocal agreements between the person's health plan and a provider in the area you will visit.

✓ If you anticipate the need for medical care, call ahead or ask your HMO to help you make doctor's appointments in the new location.

✓ Consider buying traveler's insurance. Study the policy terms regarding pre-existing conditions. READ THE FINE PRINT.

✓ Check that medical equipment is insured for loss or theft.

✓ Consider taking a portable grab bar on the trip.

- helping arrange transportation to the United States on a commercial flight (must be paid by the traveler)

- explaining various options and costs for return of remains or burial

- helping locate you, the caregiver, if you are traveling when a family member becomes ill

✓ *If traveling to a foreign country, see if the policy allows for medical evacuation.*

✓ *Take the person's health insurance card and the HMO's toll free number for travelers.*

✓ *Take copies of the pages in the insurance benefits booklet dealing with emergency access.*

✓ *Carry a card listing phone numbers of next-of-kin in case of illness during the trip.*

✓ *Carry a copy of the Consular Information Sheet of the country you are visiting.*

✓ *Write the primary care doctor's number and beeper number on the health insurance card, along with the date of the last tetanus injection.*

✓ *If taking a cruise, ask if a doctor with experience in emergency medicine or family practice will be on board.*

✓ *If the person in your care has a heart condition, check to make sure your airline carries a defibrillator in the event of cardiac arrest. Most major airlines carry them now.*

✓ *Tell the travel agent or airline that you will require a wheelchair and ask to have your request noted on the ticket.*

✓ *Call ahead to the airport, bus station or train station to request assistance.*

✓ *If a flight is delayed for more than four hours, an airline has a duty to provide a meal that is comparable to the meal offered on the flight—if asked for by the passenger.*

Travel and Living Wills

If a person becomes disabled with a life-threatening illness while traveling, the medical personnel in foreign countries may not accept the validity of an advance directive. If a person is traveling and suffers an illness that requires breathing devices or other life-prolonging treatments, it may be impossible to end the treatment without a medical evacuation back to the United States. However, there a few basic precautions you can take to ensure that a person's wishes are carried out:

- Take a copy of the living will on the trip. Let any other traveling companions know where it is packed.

- Take health-care directive documents with you.

- Consider signing the form used in the state where you might be traveling.

Choice in Dying, a nonprofit organization, has a 24-hour telephone dial-in system, called **Docudial,** that allows you to access your advance directive. Call (202) 338-9790. This organization can provide a form for an advance directive. Once the form has been completed, it (or any other form a personal attorney has drawn up) can be registered with Docudial for telephone retrieval from any location. Choice in Dying also provides a wallet-instruction card.

TRAVELING ABROAD

Tip

When traveling in tropical countries, use the standard traveler's rule: boil it, peel it, cook it, or forget it!

Travel Discount Guidelines

- The major airlines sell coupon books to those 62 and older.

- Sometimes a caregiver and the traveling companion can get the same discount.

- The companion can use the discount coupon only on the same itinerary.

- Canadian Association of Retired Persons and American Association of Retired Persons members can get at least a 10% discount in hotels.

- A senior's Medicare card can be used as identification for travel discounts.

 A common fraud is the offer of a "travel agent" ID card to qualify for discounts. The only card accepted as travel agent identification to qualify for discounts is the International Airlines Travel Agent Network (IATAN) ID card.

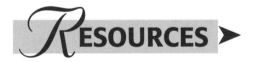 ESOURCES ►

AIDS Resources

National AIDS HOTLINE
(800) 342-AIDS (2437)
(800) 344-SIDA (Spanish) 8 a.m.–2 a.m. EST 7 days per week
(800) AIDS-889 (TTY) 10 a.m.–10 p.m. EST Monday through Friday
Operates 24 hours a day, 7 days a week and offers general information and local referrals to support groups for caregivers.

CDC National Prevention Information Network
P.O. Box 6003
Rockville, MD 20849-6003
(800) 458-5231
Fax (301)562-1001 or (888)282-7681
www.cdcnpin.org
Offers free government publications and information about resources on HIV/AIDS, STD's, and tuberculosis.

Social Security Administration
(800) SSA-1213

OR

Contact your local SS office.
Has two disability benefit programs that provide financial assistance to eligible AIDS patients.

Senior Action in a Gay Environment (SAGE)
305 7th Avenue
16th Floor
New York, NY 10001
(212) 741-2247
www.sageusa.org
Provides HIV/AIDS information and referrals for people age 50 and older.

National Institute on Aging
NIA Information Center
P.O. Box 8057
Gaithersburg, MD 20898-8057
(800) 222-2225
(800) 222-4225 (TTY)
Fax (301) 589-3014
www.nih.gov/nia
A government program that provides free publications on aging and related health issues.

Depression/Continuing Education Resources

PBS Adult Learning Service Online
www.pbs.org/learn/als

Education Index
www.educationindex.com

Comprehensive Distance Education List of Resources
www.uwex.edu/disted/websources.html

Museums of the USA
www.museumca.org/usa

SeniorNet
www.seniornet.org
An educational nonprofit organization with links to other on-line sources for older adults in the areas of government, learning, health, wellness, and other areas of interest. SeniorNet operates learning centers where seniors are taught computer skills and learn programs to access the Internet.

Administration on Aging
www.aoa.dhhs.gov
An information "ferret" with links to the Administration on Aging, Social Security Administration, National Institute of Health.

Seniors Computer Information Project
www.crm.mb.ca/scip/
A project of Creative Retirement Manitoba, this site is a guide for older adults to Manitoban, Canadian, and world-wide information and services.

National Organization for Victim Assistance (NOVA)
1730 Park Road, NW
Washington, D.C. 20010
(800) 879-6682 (TRY-NOVA) 24-hour hotline
www.try-nova.org
A nonprofit organization that provides the name and number of a victim's assistance support group in your area, and free informational brochures. They also provide training in crisis response.

Council of Better Business Bureaus
(703) 276-0100
www.bbb.org
Will refer you to the Council of Better Business Bureaus in your area, by your zip code, for the business you are inquiring about.

Healthworld Online
www.healthy.net
Web site with an orientation toward homeopathic, holistic health, and other alternative medicine.

Healthguide Online
www.healthguide.com
Web site created at the Western Psychiatric Institute of the University of Pittsburgh.

American Speech-Language-Hearing Association
10801 Rockville Pike
Rockville, MD 20852
(800) 638-8255
(301) 897-5700 (in Maryland)
www.asha.org
Provides free information on various communication disorders and makes referrals to audiologists and speech pathologists.

Pain Management Resources

American Academy of Medical Acupuncture
www.medicalacupuncture.org
Will provide the names of member acupuncturists who are also medical doctors.

The National Chronic Pain Outreach Association
P.O. Box 274
Millboro, VA 24460
(540) 862-9437
Fax: (540)862-9485
www.chronicpain.org
E-mail: ncpoa@cfw.com
A membership organization that offers a quarterly newsletter (Lifeline), a catalogue of related publications, national physician referrals, and support group listings. Membership is $25 per year.

The Worldwide Congress on Pain
http://www.pain.com

Transportation and Travel Resources

Travel Assistance International
9200 Keystone Crossing
Suite 300
Indianapolis, IN 46240
(800) 821-2828
(317) 575-2652
Fax (317)-575-2659
www.travelassistance.com
A for-profit company which provides members with worldwide, 24-hours-per-day comprehensive travel services such as on-site emergency medical payments, emergency medical transportation, and assistance with medication replacement.

Centers for Disease Control and Prevention
(877) FYI-TRIP (394-8747)
Fax requests: (888) 232-3299
www.cdc.gov
Provides recommendations on vaccinations and health data for travel to specific countries; also provides information about diseases such as malaria and yellow fever.

Consular Information Program
Bureau of Consular Affairs
State Department
(202) 647-3000 for automatic fax
(202) 647-5225 for recorded messages
www.travel.state.gov
Provides travel advisory information and emergency assistance. Ask for a complete set of Department of State, Bureau of Consular Affairs publications including "Medical Information for Americans Traveling Abroad."

Diet and Nutrition

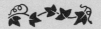

Diet and Nutrition

*P*roper nutrition is basic to good health. An older person's diet should avoid high-calorie, low-nutrient food. As the body ages, a person has to make more of an effort to eat wisely. However, there is no need to change food habits to drastically lower fat intake.

Most older people need fewer calories to maintain normal body weight. Their bodies absorb fewer nutrients so they must eat high-nutrient food to maintain good health. **They must get more nutrients from less food.** If a person does not get enough calories, the body will use stored nutrients for energy. When this happens, the person becomes weaker and is more likely to get infections.

Check with the doctor before starting any special diets, especially for the person with a swallowing impairment. Also, check with a doctor, pharmacist, or registered dietitian to know what effect prescription medicines have on nutritional needs.

> **NOTE** Use every means possible to perk up the appetite. Make sure the person's dentures fit correctly and that his or her glasses are adequate. We eat with our eyes before we ever touch our food.

Careful Food Preparation

Older people are especially susceptible to illness from unsafe food, so be extra careful when preparing their meals.

- Wash your own hands and the hands of the person in care with antibacterial soap before preparing or serving food.

- Dry hands with a paper towel.

- Disinfect the sink and kitchen counters with a solution of 1 teaspoon chlorine bleach per liter of water. (Save the solution for just one week because it loses strength.)

- Air drying dishes is more sanitary than using a dish towel.

- Check expiration dates carefully, and discard all meats that are past the expiration date on the label.

- Cook all red meat and fish thoroughly.

- Cook hamburgers or chopped meat to an *internal* temperature of 160° F. (There is much less chance of being infected by a solid piece of meat like a steak or roast because bacteria collects only on the outside of those cuts.)

- Cook meat at least at an oven temperature of 300° F.

- Keep hot foods hot at 140° F or more and cold foods at 40° F or colder.

- Keep the refrigerator below 41 degrees

- Cook eggs until the yolks are no longer runny.

- Don't serve raw eggs in milk shakes or other drinks.

- Don't serve oysters, clams, or shellfish raw.

- Wash all fruits and vegetables thoroughly.

- Avoid unpasteurized milk and cider.

 NOTE If the water temperature is set too low, the dishwasher will not sterilize the dishes.

Nutrition Guidelines for the Elderly

Be aware of any medical condition that would require restrictions such as salt (congestive heart failure) or potassium (kidney failure).

- Make tasty, nutritionally well-balanced meals that promote good bowel function and a normal flow of urine.

- Offer drinking water or liquids at mealtime to make chewing and swallowing easier.

- Avoid lard, bacon fat, coconut and palm kernel oil, sweets, and highly seasoned foods.

- Serve fresh fruits and vegetables. They are good sources of fiber and Vitamins A and C and they prevent constipation.

- Do not serve too much refined food, which lacks fiber and contributes to constipation.

- To improve sluggish appetites, use seasonings like herbs, spices, lemon juice, peppers, garlic, and vinegar, especially if salt is restricted.

Boosting Calorie or Protein Intake

- Offer most of the food when the person is most hungry.

- Encourage the person to eat food with the fingers if it increases intake.

- Add non-fat powdered milk to any food with liquid in it, such as desserts, soups, gravy, and cereal.

- Add butter, whipped cream, or sour cream to foods.

- Add cottage cheese or ricotta cheese to casseroles, scrambled eggs, and desserts.

- Grate hard cheeses on bread, meats, vegetables, eggs, and casseroles.

- Use instant breakfast powder in milk drinks and desserts.

- Add nuts, seeds, and wheat germ to breads, cereal, casseroles, and desserts.

- Add beaten eggs to mashed potatoes, sauces, vegetable purees, and cooked puddings.

- Add honey, jam, or sugar to bread, milk drinks, fruit, and yogurt desserts.

- Add mayonnaise to salads and sandwiches.

Quick and Easy Snacks

Be sure to first check with your doctor about sugar, salt, or potassium restrictions.

- buttered popcorn

- cheese on crackers

- chocolate milk

- fruits, especially ripe bananas

- granola cookies

- hard boiled eggs

- milkshakes

- puddings

- raisins, nuts, prunes

PREPARING FOOD

Tip

When preparing a meal for your family, put a small amount in the blender to make it easier for the person in your care to eat.

Therapeutic Diets

Keep the doctor informed about the diet you follow. A special diet may be prescribed to:

- improve or maintain a person's health

- change the amount of bulk, as in a high fiber diet

- change the consistency of food, as in a special soft diet

- eliminate or decrease certain foods

- change the number of calories

Dehydration Prevention

As a person ages, he feels less thirsty, so a special effort should be made to provide enough fluids. A person's fluid balance can be affected by medication, emotional stress, exercise, nourishment, general health, and the weather. Dehydration, especially in the elderly, can increase confusion and muscle weakness and cause nausea. Nausea, in turn, will prevent the person from wanting to eat, thereby causing more dehydration.

Preventative measures include:

- encouraging 6–8 cups of liquid every day (or an amount determined by the doctor)

- serving beverages at room temperature

- providing foods high in liquid (for example, watermelon)

- avoiding caffeine, which causes frequent urination and dehydration

Osteoporosis Prevention

Older people—especially women—suffer from osteoporosis, a condition that occurs when minerals are lost from the bones, thereby weakening them to the point where they break easily and are slow to heal.

Osteoporosis can be prevented by:

- getting adequate vitamin D from sunshine a few times per week, and from fortified milk (not yogurt), fatty fish, or a vitamin supplement

- getting calcium from dairy foods; leafy vegetables such as kale and collards; broccoli; salmon; and sardines

- taking calcium supplements (with vitamin C in the evening because it absorbs during sleep)

 The National Institutes of Health recommends that postmenopausal women consume 1,500 milligrams of calcium daily to slow bone loss.

Recommended Daily Allowances for a Person Over Age 51

If you are concerned that an elderly person is malnourished, do a calorie check periodically. Recommended daily allowances are:

- women—1900 calories per day (63 grams fat)

- men—2200 calories per day (73 grams fat)

Additional Sources of Protein, Calcium, and Folate

The diets of the elderly are often deficient in these nutrients which are found in the following foods: (* denotes most concentrated sources)

Calcium (one cup serving, except where noted)
Cheddar cheese (1 oz.)
Collards (1/2 cup, cooked)
Lactaid milk, nonfat, calcium fortified*
Milk, skim or 1%
Orange juice, with added calcium*
Ricotta, fat-free (1/4 cup)

Swiss cheese (1 oz.)*
Total® brand cereal (3/4 cup)*
Yogurt, nonfat, plain*

Folate (one cup serving, except where noted)
Brewer's yeast (1 tablespoon)
Chickpeas or pinto beans, cooked
Ensure brand nutrition supplement
Lentils, cooked*
Orange juice
Product 19 brand cereal*
Red kidney beans
Spinach (1/2 cup, cooked)
Total® brand cereal (3/4 cup)*

Protein (4 oz. serving, except where noted)
Beans or peas (1 cup)
Beef steak, eye of round, well trimmed*
Chicken (without skin or bone)*
Chili with beans (1 cup)
Eggs
Flounder*
Lamb, well trimmed*
Lentils (1 cup cooked)*
Pork tenderloin, well trimmed*
Salmon, canned, drained
Tuna, canned in water, drained*
Turkey (without skin or bone)*
Yogurt, nonfat, plain (8 oz.)

NOTE These may not be the best foods for a person under special medical treatment. Special diets and products to improve nutrition should only be used on the advice of a doctor or registered dietitian. If a special diet is needed due to an existing medical condition or disease, contact your local out-patient dietitian or diabetes treatment program.

Checklist **Nutrition Assessment**

To assess nutrition risk for the person in your care, check the following questions. If the answer to most of the points is Yes, the person is at risk and you need to contact the doctor for a diet. Answer the questions every six months or whenever you notice big changes in weight or eating habits.

✓ *Has she recently lost weight?* _____

   About how much? _____ *lbs.*

✓ *Has she had any recent appetite loss?* _____

   For how long? _____
   (days, weeks, months)

✓ *Does she have difficulty chewing?*
   _____

✓ *Does she have difficulty swallowing?* _____

✓ *Food allergies?* _____
   _____

✓ *A special diet?* _____

   _____
   _____
   _____

✓ *Have you been given instructions about her diet?* _____

✓ *Does she eat fewer than 2 meals per day?* _____

✓ *Does she eat few fruits, vegetables, and dairy products?*
   _____

✓ *How many servings per day?*
   Fruits _____
   Vegetables _____
   Dairy _____

✓ *Does she drink more than 3 alcoholic beverages per day?* _____

✓ *Does she eat most of her meals alone?* _____

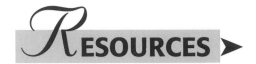

RESOURCES ➤

American Dietetic Association
(800) 366-1655
Call weekdays 10:00 a.m. to 5:00 p.m. EST to locate a registered dietitian in your area.

Area Agency on Aging or the **Cooperative Extension Service**
Your local office offers free counseling by a registered dietitian.

Meals-on-Wheels
Can provide nutritious meals delivered to the home.

Eldercare Locator
(800) 677-1116
Call to locate a Senior Nutrition Center in your area.

F.D.A. Food Safety Information Hotline
(888) SAFE FOOD (723-3366)
www.fda.gov **OR** www.cfsan.fda.gov
Offers food safety and nutrition information in English and Spanish from specialists from 10:00 a.m. to 4:00 p.m. EST; provides recorded information 24 hours a day.

U.S.D.A. Meat & Poultry Hotline
(800) 535-4555
www.fsis.usda.gov
Provides recorded messages on food safety and preparation 24 hours a day, and specialists to answer specific questions from 10:00 a.m. to 4:00 p.m. EST.

Emergencies

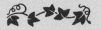

Emergencies

*E*mergency situations are common with the elderly because of their chronic illnesses and problems resulting from falls. Many injuries can be avoided through preventative measures (📖 See *Preparing the Home*, page 91) *but when a crisis does occur, use common sense, stay calm, and realize that you can help.*

> **NOTE** Make sure 911 is posted on your phone or ideally is on speed-dial, and keep written instructions on how to get to the street address of your house. If you have a speaker phone, use the speaker when talking to the dispatcher. By using the speaker phone, you can follow the dispatcher's instructions while attending to the emergency.

When to Call for an Ambulance

Call for an ambulance if a person—

- becomes unconscious

- has chest pain or pressure

- has trouble breathing

- has no signs of circulation (no breathing, no coughing, no movement)

- is bleeding severely

- is vomiting blood or is bleeding from the rectum

- has fallen and may have broken bones

- has had a seizure

- has a severe headache and slurred speech

- has pressure or severe pain in the abdomen that does not go away

OR

- moving the person could cause further injury

- traffic or distance would cause a life-threatening delay in getting to the hospital

- the person is too heavy for you to lift or help

Ambulance service is expensive and may not be covered by insurance. Use it only when you believe there is an emergency. In an emergency:

Step 1: Call 911.
Step 2: Care for the victim.

Also call 911 for emergency situations involving fire, explosion, poisonous gas, downed electrical wires, or other life-threatening emergencies.

 NOTE If the person in your care has a signed Do Not Resuscitate (DNR) order, have it available to show the paramedics. (📖 see page 87) Otherwise, they are required to initiate resuscitation. The order must go with the patient. The Do Not Resuscitate order *must* be with the patient at all times.

In the Emergency Room

Be sure you understand the instructions for care before leaving the emergency room. Call the patient's personal doctor as soon as possible and let him or her know about the emergency room care.

Bring to the emergency room—

- insurance policy numbers
- a list of medical problems
- a list of medications currently being taken
- the personal physician's name and phone number
- the name and number of a relative or friend

The following descriptions of CPR and the Heimlich Maneuver are intended only to give you an idea of how the techniques are done. We recommend that you take a course in CPR from your local American Red Cross, hospital, or other agency.

CPR (Cardio-Pulmonary Resuscitation)

- Use CPR when a person is unresponsive, is not breathing, and has no signs of circulation (normal breathing, coughing, or movements).
- Do not take more than 10 seconds to check for signs of circulation.
- If the victim does not respond after you provide the two breaths, you must begin chest compressions.
- Use Rescue Breathing (described below) if a person is not breathing but has signs of circulation (breathing, coughing, moving).
- Use a face shield (from any medical supply store) and gloves.

*If the Person Is Unresponsive, But **Has Signs of Circulation*** *(Breathing, Coughing, Moving)*

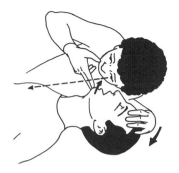

◀ *1*

- Call 911.

- Tilt the head back and lift the chin.

- Look, listen, and feel for breathing.

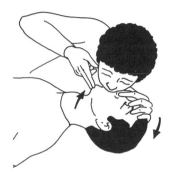

◀ *2* *If not breathing:*

- Pinch the person's nose shut, open your mouth wide, and make a tight seal around the person's mouth.

 —Give two slow breaths (2 seconds for each breath).

 —Allow for exhalation between breaths.

- Provide Rescue Breathing (1 breath every 5–6 seconds).

Signs of Circulation:
- Normal breathing
- Coughing
- Movement

◀ *3*

- Check for signs of circulation every minute.

- If there are no signs of ciculation, begin 15 chest compressions followed by two Rescue Breaths. See next page.

If A Person Is Unresponsive, And *Has No Signs of Circulation* (No Breathing, Coughing, Moving)

1
- Call 911.
- Tilt the head back and lift the chin.
- Look, listen, and feel for breathing.

2
- Pinch the person's nose shut, open your mouth wide, and make a tight seal around the person's mouth.

    —Give two slow breaths (2 seconds each).

    —Allow for exhalation between breaths.

- Provide Rescue Breathing (1 breath every 5–6 seconds).

3
- Check for a signs of circulation.

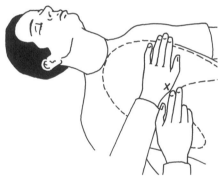

◄ *4*

- If there are no signs of circulation, begin chest compressions (15 chest compressions followed by two Rescue Breaths) at a rate of 100 times per minute. Locate the heel of one hand over the lower ⅓ of the breast bone, place the heel of the other hand on top of the hand on the breast bone.

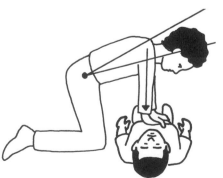

◄ *5*

- Push down on the chest about 1½ to 2 inches, 100 compressions a minute, followed by 2 slow breaths.

- After completing 4 cycles of 15 compressions and two slow breaths, check for the return of signs of circulation. If there are no signs of circulation, continue CPR.

Choking (Adult)

Prevention (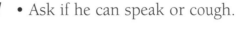 See *Eating*, page 192)

- Avoid serving excessive alcohol.

- Make sure the person in your care has a good set of dentures to chew food adequately.

- Cut the food into small pieces.

- For stroke victims, use thickening powder in liquids.

- Do not encourage the person to talk while eating.

- Do not make him laugh while eating.

If the Adult Is Choking

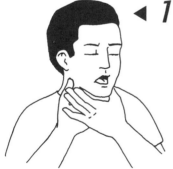

◄ *1* • Ask if he can speak or cough.

▼*2* • If the person CANNOT SPEAK, give abdominal thrusts (the Heimlich Maneuver). Stand behind the person, place your fist just above the navel, clasp your fist with the other hand, and give quick, upward thrusts until the object is removed or the person becomes unconscious.

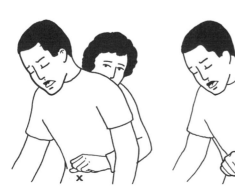

3 If the person becomes **unconscious,** lower him to the floor onto his back.

4 Call 911.

5 Tilt the head back and lift the chin to open the airway. Sweep the mouth with your fingers to remove any objects.

6 Place your mouth over the victim's and try to give 2 breaths. Reposition the head if necessary and try to give two more breaths.

7 Repeat Steps 5 and 6 until help arrives.

OR

- If breathing starts, place the person on his side in the **RECOVERY POSITION.** (See illustration, below.)

▶ *Placing person in the Recovery Position*

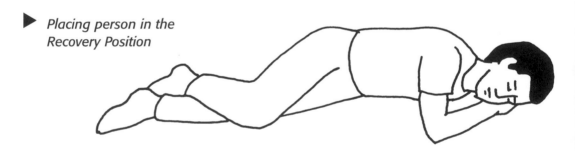

Bleeding

If someone is bleeding heavily, protect yourself with rubber gloves, plastic wrap, or layers of cloth. Then—

1. Apply direct pressure over the wound with a clean cloth.

2. Apply another clean cloth on top of the blood-soaked cloth, keeping the pressure firm.

3. If no bones are broken, elevate the injured limb to decrease blood flow.

4. Call 911 for an ambulance.

5. Apply a bandage snugly over the dressing.

6. Wash your hands with soap and water as soon as possible after providing care.

7. Avoid contact with blood-soaked objects.

Shock

Shock may be associated with heavy bleeding, hives, shortness of breath, dizziness, swelling, thirst, and chest pain. The signs of shock are:

- restlessness and irritability

- altered consciousness, confusion

- pale, cool, moist skin

- rapid breathing and weakness

If these signs are present—

1. Have the person lie down.

2. Control any bleeding.

3. Keep the person warm.

4. Elevate the legs about 12-14 inches unless the neck or back has been injured.

5. Do not give the person anything to eat or drink.

6. Call 911.

Burns

1. Stop the burning process by pouring large amounts of cold water over the burn.

2. Do *not* remove clothing stuck to the burned area.

3. Cover the burn with a dry, clean covering.

4. Keep the person warm.

5. For **chemical burns to the eyes,** flush them with large amounts of cool running water (faucet or shower).

OR

Immerse the face in water and have the person open and close his eyes.

6. Call 911 for transport to hospital.

Chest Pain

Any chest pain that lasts more than a few minutes is related to the heart until proven otherwise. Call 911 immediately. Don't wait to see if it goes away. Danger signs include—

• pain radiating from the chest down the arms, up the neck to the jaw, and into the back

• crushing, squeezing chest pain or heavy pressure in the chest

- shortness of breath, sweating, nausea and vomiting, weakness

- bluish, pale skin

- skin that is moist

- excessive perspiration

If the person is not breathing, begin Rescue Breathing, and check for signs of circulation (breathing, coughing, moving). (📖 See # 1, #2, #3 on page 251.)

If there is no signs of circulation, begin CPR. (📖 See page 252.)

Falls and Related Injuries

Falls are common in the elderly. The high risk times are during an illness, after using the toilet, immediately after eating (drinking tea or coffee after a meal may counteract this), and immediately after sitting up.

Preventative measures include:

- staying in when it is rainy or icy outside

- having regular vision screening check-ups for correct eye glasses

- using separate reading glasses and other regular glasses if bifocals make seeing the floor difficult

- being cautious when walking on wet floors

- wearing good foot support when walking

- being aware that new shoes are slippery and crepe soled shoes can cause the toe to catch

- having foot pain problems corrected

- keeping toenails trimmed and feet healthy for good balance

A good way to tell if a part of the body has been injured in a fall is to compare it with an uninjured part. For example, compare the injured leg with the uninjured leg. Do they look and feel the same? Do they move the same way?

When you suspect a **broken bone,** follow these steps:

- If the person **cannot** move or use the injured limb, keep it from moving. Do not straighten a deformed arm or leg. Splint an injury in the position you find it.

- Support the injured part above and below the site of the injury by using folded towels, blankets, pillows, or magazines.

- If the person is face down, roll him over with the "log rolling" technique (See below). If you have no one to help you and the victim is breathing adequately, leave the person in the same position.

- If the person does not complain of neck pain but is feeling sick to his stomach, turn him on one side.

- If the person complains of neck pain, keep his neck steady by putting a few pillows on either side of his head. Keep the head flat.

- Apply ice to the injury site, over a piece of cloth.

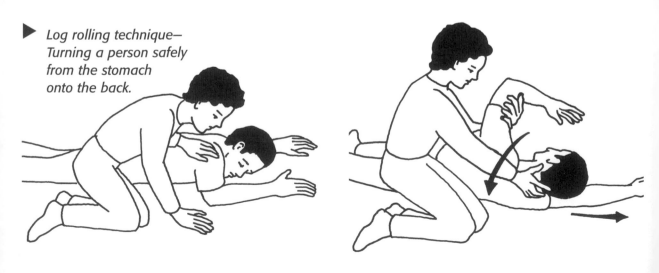

▶ *Log rolling technique— Turning a person safely from the stomach onto the back.*

- Keep the person warm with a blanket and make him as comfortable as possible.

- Make a splint with cardboard or rolled-up newspaper.

 If an arm or shoulder is splinted, transport the person by car. For neck, hip, thigh, back, and pelvic injuries, use an ambulance because the person needs to lie flat.

Fainting

Fainting can be caused by—

- heart attacks

- medications

- low blood sugar

- standing up quickly

- straining to have a bowel movement

- dehydration

To some extent, fainting can be prevented.

- Ask the doctor if medications that do not cause fainting can be prescribed.

- Monitor blood sugar levels.

- Avoid constipation.

- Do not let the person stand up or sit up too rapidly.

If a fainting spell occurs:
1. Do not try to place the person in a sitting position. Instead, immediately lay him down flat.

2. Check the person's airway, breathing, and pulse.

3. Turn him on his side.

4. Elevate the legs.

5. Cover him with a blanket if the room or floor is cold.

6. Do not force fluids.

7. Use CPR if necessary (📖 See page 252).

Hypothermia

Hypothermia occurs when a person's body temperature falls below normal (98.6° F). Conditions that may alter the person's body response to cold are:

- hypothyroidism

- arthritis

- dizziness and resulting falls

- excessive alcohol

- stroke

- head injuries

- medications that cause poor temperature regulation

To prevent hypothermia—

- Keep the house temperature no lower than 65° F (at 70° F if the person is ill).

- Have him wear warm clothes, and place wool leg warmers on his arms and legs for extra warmth.

- Use warm blankets when the person is in bed.

- Wear a warm hat outside or a knit hat to keep the body from losing heat indoors.

• Provide a balanced diet.

• Provide exercise of some sort.

Signs of hypothermia include impaired judgment, shivering, cold pale skin, slow breathing and pulse, weakness, drowsiness, and confusion. If these signs are present:

1. Wrap the person in blankets, notify the doctor, give warm fluids, and increase room temperature.

2. Avoid rubbing the person's skin.

3. Do not rewarm the person rapidly. Use a heater on low or warm hot water bottles on the chest and abdomen.

4. Do not give the person alcohol.

5. Be alert to signs of heart attack (📖 See page 256.)

Heat Stroke

An older person is at greater risk of heat stroke because the aging body is less able to cool itself. Also, some medications can increase the likelihood it will occur and the elderly may not feel the heat. To prevent heat stroke—

• Ask the doctor if the medicine the person is taking can increase the risk of heat stroke.

• Use clothing made of breathable lightweight fabrics.

• Use a fan, damp compresses, or an air conditioner.

• Have the person drink 6–8 glasses of water even if she is not feeling thirsty. (📖 See *Dehydration,* page 242.)

• Avoid alcohol, caffeine, and smoking because they speed dehydration.

- Avoid activity during the hottest part of the day.

Signs of heat stroke include headache, nausea, and sudden dizziness. Consult the doctor immediately to determine whether it is a serious condition.

Poisons

When you suspect poisoning, immediately take these steps:
1. Determine **what** was swallowed, **how much,** and at **what time.**

2. Check the person's airway, breathing, and pulse.

3. Contact the nearest Poison Control Center for treatment; have the container of the suspected poison at hand.

4. Contact the doctor.

5. If necessary, start CPR.

6. If necessary, call 911 for transport to the hospital.

Seizures

A seizure usually lasts from 1 to 5 minutes. If it lasts longer than 7 minutes, call 911 for an ambulance.
1. Remove all objects that might cause the person to injure himself.

2. Place pillows and blankets around him to protect him.

3. *Do **not** hold or restrain the person.

4. *Do **not** place anything in his mouth.

5. Always check for **breathing** and **signs of circulation** after the seizure stops.

6. If the person is not breathing, administer Rescue Breathing and check for signs of circulation (breathing, coughing, moving) frequently (See page 251).

7. If there are *no signs of circulation,* compress the chest 15 times, followed by 2 slow Rescue Breaths.

8. Call 911.

9. Continue CPR until help arrives.

Stroke

Strokes occur when the blood flow to the brain is interrupted by a clogged or burst blood vessel. Strokes cannot always be prevented, but the chances of their occurring can be lessened through—

- a balanced diet

- avoidance of stress

- periodic checkups

- regular exercise

- regular use of a prescribed blood pressure medicine

Suspect a stroke when the person in your care—

- has a sudden and severe headache

- is not responsive to simple statements

- has a seizure

- is suddenly incontinent

- has paralysis in an arm or leg

- cannot grip equally with both hands

- appears droopy on one side of the face

- has slurred speech or blurred vision

- is confused

- has an unsteady gait

- has trouble swallowing

- has loss of balance or coordination when combined with another sign

The chance of recovery from a stroke is markedly increased if the victim has immediate help.

1. Keep the person in the position you found him in.

2. Reassure him and keep him calm.

3. If he has trouble breathing, open his airway, tilt his head, lift his chin.

4. Check for signs of circulation (breathing, coughing, moving).

5. If the person is not breathing, give 2 Rescue Breaths.

6. If breathing resumes, place the person on one side to prevent choking and to help keep his tongue out of his airway.

7. Call 911. Get the person to medical care as soon as possible.

Checklist **Home First Aid Kit**

Buy or make a home first aid kit. Note on the box the date when the item was purchased. Check and replenish your supplies at least once a year. They should include:

✓ *antibiotic ointment*

✓ *Band-Aids®*

✓ *disinfectant for cleaning wounds*

✓ *eye pads*

✓ *instant ice packs*

✓ *latex gloves*

✓ *roller gauze and elastic bandages*

✓ *scissors*

✓ *sterile gauze bandages (nonstick 4"x4")*

✓ *syrup of ipecac*

✓ *thermometer*

✓ *tongue depressors*

✓ *three-ounce rubber bulb to rinse out wounds*

✓ *triangle bandage*

✓ *tweezers and needle*

✓ *emergency telephone numbers*

Body Mechanics—Positioning, Moving, and Transfers

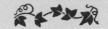

Body Mechanics—Positioning, Moving, and Transfers

Body Mechanics for the Caregiver

Body mechanics involves standing and moving one's body so as to prevent injury, avoid fatigue, and make the best use of strength. When you learn how to control and balance your own body, you can safely control and move another person. Back injuries to nursing home aides are common, so when doing any lifting be sure to use proper body mechanics.

General Rules

- Never lift more than you can comfortably handle.

- Create a base of support by standing with your feet 8-12" (shoulder width) apart with one foot a half step ahead of the other.

Proper foot position ▶

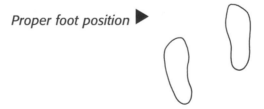

- DO NOT let your back do the heavy work—USE YOUR LEGS. (The back muscles are not your strongest muscles.)

- If the bed is low, put one foot on a foot stool. This relieves pressure on your lower back.

- Consider using a back support belt.

Helpful Caregiver Advice For Moving a Person

These pointers are for the *caregiver* only. Be sure to see the following pages for the steps for a specific move or transfer.

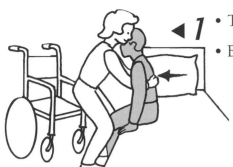

◀ **1**
- Tell the person what you are going to do.

- Before starting a move, count with the person, "1-2-3."

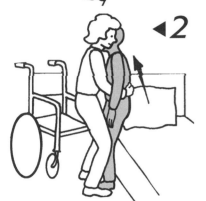

◀ **2**
- To feel in control, get close to the person you are lifting.

- While lifting, keep your back in a neutral (normal arched, not stiff) position, knees bent, weight balanced on both feet. Tighten your stomach and back muscles to maintain a correct support position.

- Use your arms to support the person.

- Again, *let your legs do the lifting.*

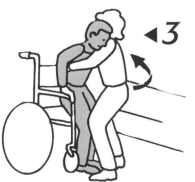

◀ **3**
- Pivot instead of twisting your body.

- Breathe deeply.

- Keep your shoulders relaxed.

- When needing to give a lot of assistance with transfers, tie a strong belt or a transfer belt around the person's waist and hold it as you complete the transfer.

Prevention of Back and Neck Injuries

To prevent injuries to yourself, get plenty of rest and maintain:

- good nutrition

- physical fitness

- good body mechanics

- a stress management program

Common Treatments for Caregiver Back Pain

If you *do* experience back pain:

- Apply a cold ice pack to the injured area for 10 minutes every hour (you can use bag of frozen vegetables).

- Get short rest periods in a comfortable position.

- With your feet shoulder width apart and hands on hips, bend backwards. Do 3–5 repetitions several times a day.

- Take short, frequent, walks on a level surface.

- Avoid sitting for long periods, because sitting is one of the worst healing positions.

As the caregiver, you should seek training from a physical therapist to provide this type of care so as to reduce the risk of injury to yourself or the person in your care. The therapist will correct any mistakes you make and can take into account special problems. To determine the best procedure for you to use, the therapist will consider the physical condition of the person you care for and the furniture and room arrangements in the home.

Moving a Person

When you have to move someone—either in bed or out of bed—remember these tips:

- Plan the move and know what you can and cannot do.

- Let the person do as much work as he is capable of.

- Always direct the activity instead of asking if the person wants to do it. Remember that your body language conveys more meaning than your words.

- Avoid letting the person put his arms around your neck or grab you.

- Use a transfer belt to balance and support the person.

- Place transfer surfaces (wheelchair and bed) close together.

- Check wheelchair position, **brakes locked,** armrests and footrests swung out of the way.

- Let the person look to the place where he is being transferred.

- If the person is able, place his hands on the bed or chair so he can assist in the movement. If the person is a stroke patient or is afraid, have him clasp his hands close to his chest.

- Ask the person to *push* rather than *pull* on the bed rails, the chair, or you.

- Work at the person's level and speed and check for pain.

- Avoid sudden jerking motions.

- Never pull on the person's arms or shoulders.

- Correctly position the person. (This helps the body regain lost function and helps prevent additional function loss.)

- Have the person to be transferred wear either shoes with good treads or sturdy slippers.

NOTE To encourage independence, let the person make a few attempts at helping. It's okay for him to stand up partly and sit back down.

Positioning a Person in Bed

1▶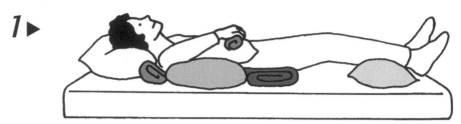

- Place a small pillow under the person's head, keeping his spine neutral.

- Place a small pillow lengthwise under the calf of the weak leg, let the heel hang off the end of the pillow to prevent pressure, and loosen the top sheet to avoid pressure on the toes.

2▶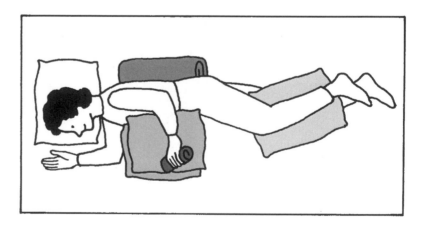

- Fold a bath towel under the hip of the person's weak side.

- Place the weak arm and elbow on a pillow higher than the heart.

Positioning a Person on His or Her Strong Side

1. Place a small pillow under the person's head.

2. Keep the person's head in alignment with the spine.

3. Place a rolled pillow at the back to prevent rolling.

4. Place a pillow in front to keep the arm the same height as the shoulder joint.

5. Place a medium pillow lengthwise between the knees, legs, and ankles. (The person's knees may be bent slightly.)

Positioning a Person on His or Her Weak Side

1. Use the same positioning as described above.

2. Change the person's position frequently because he may not be aware of pressure, pain, or skin irritation.

Moving a person in bed can injure the person in care or the caregiver if certain basic rules are not followed:

- Never grab or pull the person's arm or leg.

- If the medical condition allows, raise the foot of the bed slightly to prevent the person from sliding down.

- If moving him is difficult, get him out of bed and back in the wheelchair and start over by putting him in bed closer to the headboard.

Moving a Person Up in Bed

1. Tell the person what you are going to do.

2. Lower the head of the bed flat and remove the pillow— never try to move the person uphill.

3. If possible, raise the bed and **lock the wheels.**

4. Tell the person to bend his knees and brace his feet firmly against the mattress to help push.

5. Stand at the side of the bed and place one hand behind the person's back and the other underneath the buttocks.

6. Bend your knees and keep your back in a neutral position.

7. Count "1-2-3" and have the person push with his feet and pull with his hands toward the head of the bed.

8. Replace the pillow under his head.

Using Two People to Move an Unconscious Person

1
- Tell the person what you are going to do even if he seems unconscious.
- Remove the pillow.
- If possible, raise the bed and **lock the wheels.**

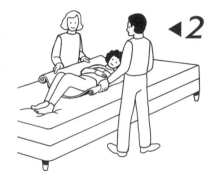

◄**2**
- Stand on either side of the bed.
- Face the head of the bed, feet 8-12" apart, knees bent, back in a neutral position.
- Roll the sides of the draw sheet up to the person's body.

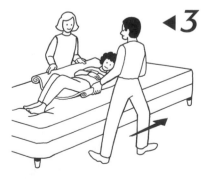

◄**3**
- Grab the draw sheet with your palms up.
- Count "1-2-3" and then shift your body weight from the back to the front leg, keeping your arms and back in a locked position and together slide the person smoothly up the bed.
- Replace pillows under the person's head.
- Position the person comfortably.

A draw sheet—a sheet folded several times and positioned under the person to be moved in bed—prevents irritation to his skin. The sheet should be positioned from the shoulders to just below the knees.

Moving an Unconscious Person Alone

1. If possible, raise the whole bed and **lock the wheels.**

2. Remove the pillow.

3. Face the front of the bed, feet 8-12" apart, knees bent, back in neutral.

4. Roll the edge of the draw sheet and grab it.

5. Slide your arms under the draw sheet and the person's shoulders and back.

6. Count "1-2-3" and then shift your body weight from your back to front leg, keeping your arms and back in a locked position.

7. Slide the person to the top of the bed.

8. Replace the pillow.

9. Position the person comfortably.

PREVENTING BACK INJURIES

Having the person grab a trapeze to help with the move is easiest and safest for your back. (See page 121.)

Moving the Person to One Side of the Bed on His or Her Back

1 • Place your feet 8–12" apart, knees bent, back in neutral.

• Slide your arms under the person's back to her far shoulder blade (bend your knees and hips to lower yourself to the person's level).

• Slide the person's shoulders toward you by rocking your weight to your back foot.

2 • Use the same procedure at the person's buttocks and feet.

• Always keep your knees bent and your back in a neutral position.

1▼

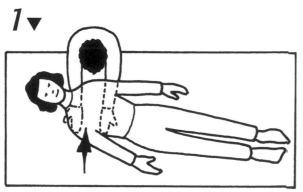

2▼

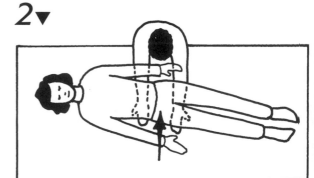

Moving the person

Rolling Technique

1. Move the person to one side of the bed as in the above procedure.

2. Bend the person's knees.

3. Hold the person at her hip and shoulder blade on the far side of the body.

4. Roll the person *toward* you to make sure she does not fall off the bed.

Raising the Person's Head and Shoulders

1. If possible, ask the person to lift her head and dig both elbows into the bed to support her body.

2. Face the head of the bed, feet 8–12" apart, knees bent, back in neutral.

3. Help the person lift her shoulders by placing your hands and forearms under the pillow and her shoulder blades.

4. Use bent knees, back in neutral, and locked arms to assist the lift.

5. Adjust the pillow.

Helping a Person Sit Up

1. Tell the person what you are going to do.

2. Bend the person's knees.

3. Roll her on her side so she is facing you.

4. Reach one arm under her shoulder blade.

5. Place the other arm in back of her knees.

6. Position your feet 8–12" apart with your center of gravity close to the bed and person.

7. Keep your back in a neutral position.

8. Count "1-2-3" and shift your weight to your back leg.

9. Shift the person's legs over the edge of the bed while pulling her shoulders to a sitting position.

10. Remain in front of her until she is stabilized.

Transfers

Transferring a person in and out of bed is an important caregiver activity, which can be accomplished with a fair degree of ease if these instructions are followed. Use the same procedure for all transfers so a routine is set up.

Transfers Using a Mechanical Lift

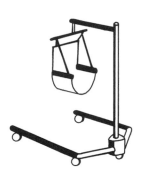

1. Tell the person what you are going to do.

2. Place the chair next to the bed with the back of the chair in line with the headboard of the bed. **Lock the wheels.**

3. Place a blanket or sheet over the chair.

4. Turn the person on one side toward the edge of the bed.

5. Fan-fold a sling and place it at the person's back.

6. Roll her to the other side, pull the sling out flat, and center it under her body.

7. Attach the sling to the mechanical lift with the hooks in place and facing out through the metal frame.

8. Fold the person's arms across his chest.

9. Using the crank, lift her out of bed.

10. Guide her legs. Lower her onto the chair.

12. Remove the hooks from the frame of the mechanical lift.

13. Leave the person in the chair with the sling under her, comfortably adjusted.

14. To get the person back in the bed, put the hooks facing out through the metal frame of the sling.

15. Raise the person using the crank.

16. Guide her legs. Lower her onto the bed.

18. Remove the hooks from the frame.

19. Remove the sling from under the person by turning her from side to side on the bed.

20. Properly position her with pillows. (See page 272.)

For lift instructions and precautions, refer to the *Positioning and Transfer Guide* that comes with your mechanical lift.

Helping a Person Stand

Help only as much as needed but guard the person from falling.

1. Have her sit on the edge of the chair or bed. Let her rest a moment in case she feels lightheaded.

2. Instruct her to push off with her hands from the bed or chair armrests.

3. Position your knee between her knees.

4. Face her and support the weak knee against one or both of your knees as needed.

5. Put your arms around the person's waist or use a transfer belt.

6. Keep your back in a neutral position.

7. At the count of "1-2-3," instruct the person to stand up while pulling her toward you and pushing your knees into her knee if needed.

8. Once she is upright, have her keep her knee locked straight.

9. Support and balance her as needed.

NOTE If during a transfer you start to "lose" the person, do not try to hold her up. Instead, lower her to the floor.

Helping a Person Sit

1. Reverse the process described above.

2. Direct the person to feel for the chair or bed with the back of the legs.

3. Direct the person to reach back with both hands to the bed or chair armrests and slowly sit.

Transferring from Bed to Wheelchair With a Transfer Belt

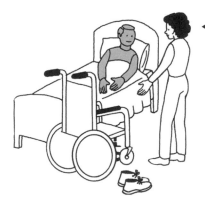

◀ *1*
- Place the wheelchair at a 45° angle to the bed so that the person will be transferring to his stronger side.

- **Lock the wheels** of the chair and the bed.

- Tell the person what you are going to do.

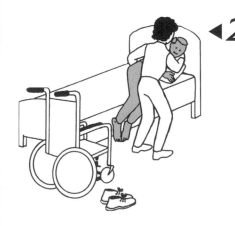

◀*2*
- Put on his shoes while he is still lying down if he is weak or unstable.

- Bring him to sitting position with his legs over the edge of the bed.

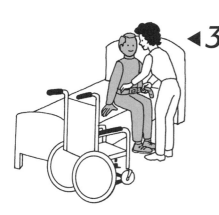

◄3
- Let him rest a moment in case he feels lightheaded.
- Use a **transfer belt** for a person needing a lot of support.

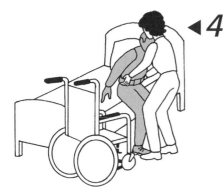

◄4
- Bring him to a standing position as described on page 279.

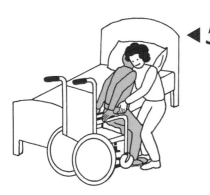

◄5
- Have him reach for the chair arm and pivot. A very fast pivot may frighten an elderly or confused person—or cause you to lose knee control and fall with a totally dependent person.
- Support him with your arms and knees as needed.
- Adjust him comfortably in the chair.

NOTE If the person starts to slide off the edge of the bed before or after the transfer, lay his upper torso across the bed to prevent him from falling to the floor.

Transferring from Wheelchair to Bed

1. Reverse the process described in the preceding page.

2. Place the chair at a 45° angle to the bed so the person is on his stronger side. **Lock the wheels.**

3. Get into a position to provide a good base of support; use good body mechanics.

4. Have the person stand, reach for the bed, and pivot.

5. Support and guide him as needed.

6. Adjust the person in bed with pillows.

Transferring from Bed to Wheelchair Without a Transfer Belt

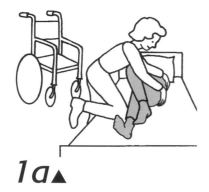

1a▲

- Place the wheelchair at a 45° angle to the bed so that the person will be transferring to his stronger side.

- **Lock the wheels** of the chair (you can use a wheel block) and the wheels of the bed.

- Tell the person what you are going to do.

- Bring him to a sitting position with his legs over the edge of the bed following steps a, b, c, and d.

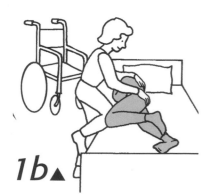

1b▲

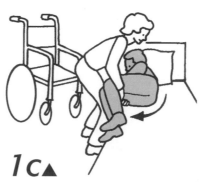

1c▲

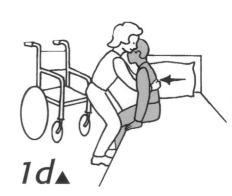

1d▲

- Let him rest a moment in case he feels lightheaded.

- Put his shoes on.

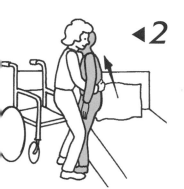

◀**2**

- Put your arms around his chest and clasp your hands behind his back.

- Support the leg that is farther from the wheelchair between your legs.

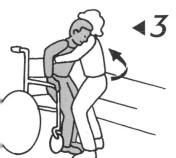

◀**3**

- Lean back, shift your leg, and lift.

- Pivot toward the chair.

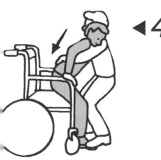

◀**4**

- Bend your knees and let the person bend toward you.

- Lower the person into the wheelchair.

- Adjust him comfortably in the chair.

NOTE As the person becomes stronger, you can provide less assistance; however, use the same body positioning to support the person's weaker side.

Transferring from Wheelchair to Bed with a Transfer Board

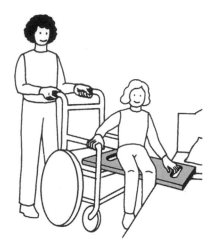

1. As much as possible, make the bed and the chair the same height.

2. Place the wheelchair at a 45° angle to the bed so that the person will be transferring to her stronger side.

3. **Lock the wheels** of the chair (you can use a wheel block) and the wheels of the bed.

4. Tell the person what you are going to do.

5. Remove the armrest nearest the bed.

6. Remove her feet from the footrests and swing the footrests out of the way.

7. Have the person lift her hip and place the board under her hip with the other end of the board on the bed.

8. BE SURE SHE DOESN'T PUT HER FINGERS UNDER THE BOARD.

9. Ask her to put her hands on the board with her hands close to her sides.

10. Ask her to lean slightly forward and to make a series of small pushes off the board by straightening her elbows and inching along the board toward the bed.

11. When she is on the bed, ask her to lean over onto her elbow and pull the transfer board out from under her bottom.

12. Adjust her comfortably in the bed.

Transferring from a Wheelchair to a Car

Be sure the car is parked on a level surface without cracks or potholes.

1
- Open the passenger door as far as possible.

- Move the left side of the wheelchair as close to the car seat as possible.

- **Lock the chair's wheels.**

- Move both footrests out of the way.

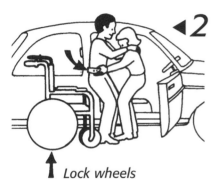

↑ *Lock wheels*

◄*2*
- Position yourself facing the person.

- Tell him what you are going to do.

- Bending your knees and hips, lower yourself to his level.

- By grasping the transfer belt around his waist help him stand while straightening your hips and knees.

- If his legs are weak, brace his knees with your knees.

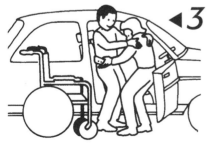

◄*3*
- While he is standing, turn him so he can be eased down to sit on the car seat. GUIDE HIS HEAD so it is not bumped.

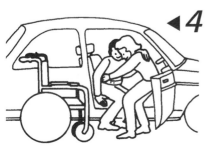

◄*4*
- Lift his legs into the car by putting your hands under his knees.

- Move him to face the front.

- Put on his seat belt.

- Close door carefully.

Understanding Dementia and Alzheimer's Disease

Dementia and Alzheimer's Disease

*D*ementia is a term used to describe the symptoms of several diseases and conditions that cause people to lose their intellectual functions. These diseases include Parkinson's, Huntington's disease, Pick's disease, AIDS, Lou Gehrig's disease, Creutzfeldt-Jacob disease, and multiple sclerosis. Of all the disorders that fall into this category, Alzheimer's disease is by far the best known. A person suffering from dementia may experience memory loss and changes in behavior—including changes in temperament, judgment, and interactions with others.

However, many people who begin to exhibit signs of memory loss and confusion are not suffering from dementia or Alzheimer's. Rather, their symptoms may stem from depression, stress, malnutrition, the side effects of several medications, vitamin deficiencies, strokes, epilepsy, untreated urinary tract infection (in women) or other factors—some of which can be easily corrected.

Anyone suspected of having dementia should have a full geriatric assessment to determine the cause of the confusion. Teaching hospitals generally have a geriatric assessment clinic. Call the local Area Agency on Aging for the nearest assessment clinic.

What Is Alzheimer's Disease?

According to the Alzheimer's Association, Alzheimer's disease, which affects 4 million Americans, is a "progressive, degenerative disease that attacks the brain." Alzheimer's patients have blockages in the areas of the brain that deal with intellectual functions and memory. In addition, they lack a vital brain chemical needed to process memory.

Alzheimer's strikes brilliant minds and average minds. Although symptoms vary, those who are afflicted cannot control their behavior and exhibit personality changes. To date, Alzheimer's cannot be cured, but drugs to reduce symptoms can be prescribed.

People with Alzheimer's become terrified because they don't understand what is happening to them. When caring for a confused person it is very important to view the situation from that person's perspective and to be aware of the terror that he or she is feeling.

 Seniors with Alzheimer's are able to live at home longer when their spouses get counseling and join support groups. Spouse caregivers need a lot of support and assistance to keep their loved one at home.

Symptoms of Alzheimer's

Some of the warning signs that Alzheimer's may be present are:

- loss of memory

- decreased attention span

- decreased ability to learn

- loss of ability to recall the appropriate word or phrase

- loss of thinking ability, judgment, and decision making

- disorientation and trouble finding the way home or to the bathroom

- loss of mathematical ability

- loss of coordination

- changes in personality

- loss of initiative, indifference

- changes in emotion—especially increased depression and agitation

Stages of Alzheimer's Disease

Once Alzheimer's begins, it passes through four fairly distinct stages.

Beginning Stage

- difficulty with balancing a check book

- forgetfulness and absentmindedness (paying the same bill twice)

- fatigue

- inability to recall common words

- a tendency to replace forgotten words with different words

- a tendency to lose track of a conversation and ramble

- inappropriate social behavior

Middle Stage

- decreased motor ability

- decreased memory

- loss of logic

- pacing and wandering

- an inability to be patient

- a tendency to strike out verbally

- deteriorating social skills

- paranoia
- aggressive behavior
- resistance to offers of help
- a need to be reminded to go to the toilet
- a decreased attention span
- increased confusion and disorientation
- decreased word recall and recognition
- increased trouble following directions
- a resistance to having anyone but the primary caregiver in the home
- a desire to have the caregiver in sight at all times

Advanced Stage

- inability to be reached intellectually
- inability to communicate
- loss of bowel and bladder control
- a tendency to have hallucinations (for example, to believe that people on TV are in the room)
- a tendency to be emotionally unresponsive
- a tendency to groan or scream and try to suck on things

Final Stage

- loss of all memory—failure to recognize family members or even one's own image in the mirror
- loss of all speech and motor coordination, including the memory of how to chew and swallow

- loss of all intellectual abilities

- inability to understand or remember what is happening

- a tendency to scream spontaneously or to be mute

The Most Difficult Symptoms for the Alzheimer's Afflicted Person

- frustration at losing the ability to communicate

- pain and embarrassment over the loss of ability to recall family members and friends

- difficulty with common tasks like dressing

- loss of independence

- forced immobility

- awareness of memory changes

The Most Difficult Symptoms for the Caregiver

- the person's inability to follow instructions and perform daily tasks

- repetition of phrases or stories

- wandering

- rage, withdrawal, and use of profanity

- demands to do things (like driving) that are no longer safe

- public displays of sexuality (exposing oneself, touching oneself inappropriately in public, initiating sexual advances with a family member who looks like the person's spouse did at the same age)

Loss of Communication Skills

Stages

The ability to communicate decreases in each stage:

Stage 1

- Because of forgotten words, long pauses occur between words and sentences.

- Forgotten words are replaced with different words.

- The person loses track of the subject and rambles.

Stage 2

- The attention span decreases.

- Confusion and disorientation increase.

- Word recall and recognition decrease.

- The ability to follow directions decreases.

Stage 3

- It is not possible to reach the person's intellect.

- All ability to communicate is lost.

In Stage 3, you can continue to speak to the person softly and maintain eye contact. Smile warmly and often. The person with Alzheimer's easily picks up on your mood. Also make sure the person has proper glasses or a hearing aid. A skilled audiologist can suggest listening devices for a confused person.

> **NOTE** Alzheimer's can erase all memory of a person's second language so the person reverts to the language spoken in childhood.

Improving Communication

Learning how to communicate with the person with Alzheimer's is very important. The person has his own reality so **do not try to reason with him**. Your manner, and the calming techniques you use, can have a positive effect. Try to respond to the *emotion*—not the *behavior*.

Improving Your Chances of Being Understood

- Reduce background noise. (When household sounds are magnified and distorted, they can cause pain and stress to the nervous system.)

- Make sure the person has proper glasses or a hearing aid.

- Get the person's attention by lightly touching an arm.

- Communicate at the person's height.

- Address the person by name and remind him of your name.

- Use a quiet, relaxed, warm approach and explain what you are going to do before you do it. This minimizes the risk of upset.

- Bend to eye level and establish eye contact.

- Speak in the person's native tongue.

- Use a soft, soothing tone of voice.

- Be a good listener and read eye and body language.

- Speak in short, direct sentences using one-step commands, pointing to the object you are discussing.

- Repeat or rephrase as necessary.

- Point to the objects you are discussing and use names for clarity. For example, say "Do you want your slippers?" not "Do you want these?"

- Write the thought you are communicating in large block letters.

- Change your patterns of communication that are disturbing, because the person's ability to communicate can be further impaired by stress.

- Avoid expressions such as "Jump into bed" that can be taken literally. They may cause unnecessary confusion.

Maintaining a Calm Atmosphere

Maintain an atmosphere of slow movement and low stimulation. Television programs should be quiet and non-violent, all beverages should be caffeine-free, and family arguments should be avoided.

- Develop a consistent routine of care.

- Offer something to hold, or a pet to stroke, or your arm to hold on to.

- Be sensitive to changing moods and do not take them personally.

- Accept the person's version of a situation. **Do not argue.**

- Tell the person when you are leaving the room.

- For any non-critical situation, do not insist on immediate treatment, but wait until the person relaxes.

- For an important treatment say, "This is for your protection," and proceed without arguing.

- Be aware that a person who is unable to describe what he wants may get very excited and start banging on furniture. When this happens, ask obvious questions first to find out what the need or concern might be.

- In cases of memory loss, reassure the person by stating who you are.

- Avoid asking confusing or embarrassing questions.

- Offer reassurance and comfort.

- Apologize.

- Use humor.

- Say the person's name softly.

- If the person expresses a desire to "go home," explain that "You are home."

- Reassure the person that his children are safe.

- Show affection and offer praise.

- Pray with the person.

- Kiss or hug him.

- Rub his back.

- Distract the person with stories about people he once knew.

 NOTE Remember—The person with Alzheimer's is very sensitive to your moods and body language, even when he doesn't understand what you say.

Relieving Boredom

Boredom in Alzheimer's patients can lead to restlessness and agitation. Finding the right activities to keep the person occupied and stimulated is a challenging task. Recognizing that the person's preferences and abilities will change over the course of the disease, try these activities:

- doing things the person enjoyed before becoming ill

- gardening

- going for a ride or walk

- attending religious services

- attending specialized programs at adult day-care centers

- watching television (if the person does not become confused or anxious)

- playing music from a favorite era

- socializing with friends

- setting up a desk with papers so the person can do "work" and keep an appointment book

- setting up a safe workbench with tools

Find ways to relieve boredom (folding laundry, tearing rags, clipping coupons, stacking cups, rolling skeins of yarn, sorting buttons, wrapping things with toilet tissue, sanding wood, dusting, sweeping the floor, typing, setting the table).

Have someone call the person on the telephone to serve as a link to the outside world.

Special Challenges

The symptoms of Alzheimer's are difficult for the patient and the caregiver to deal with. Here are some of the things to be aware of.

Symptoms of Agitation from Brain Damage Due to Injury, Stroke, or Illness

- disorientation

- extreme fear

- grabbing at bedrails for fear of falling

- hallucinations

- convulsive jerking

- kicking

- lashing out with fists

- shaking

- uncontrollable violent motion

The caregiver can cope by:

- avoiding the person's blows and kicks

- administering doctor-prescribed tranquilizers

- toileting every two hours

- reassuring the person in a calm voice

- using a restraint (posey) for safety in bed

- keeping the sides of the bed in their "up" position

- keeping the bed in the low position or putting the mattress on the floor

How to Deal with Hallucinations or Delusions

- Ignore the hallucination if it isn't frightening the person.

- Avoid contradicting or upsetting him.

- Offer reassurance about these fears.

- Recognize the person's emotions.

- Try reassuring statements.

- In severe cases, ask the doctor to prescribe medication.

Sundown Syndrome

Sundown Syndrome is a condition that involves disruptive and unusual behaviors, such as severe confusion, pacing, confused language, and paranoia, in the late afternoon and early evening. The behavior can be caused by too much excitement during the day, excess energy from lack of exercise, and strange shadows and colors at sunset. To help manage the behavior:

- Develop a consistent routine.

- Limit bathing to the morning to avoid over-stimulation.

- Arrange for a rest time during the day.

- Avoid outside visitors after 5 p.m.

- Be sure glasses and hearing aides are adequate and in place.

- Provide adequate nutrition.

- Eliminate sugar and caffeine after 5 p.m.

- Provide adequate opportunities for exercise.

- Turn on lights and close window blinds to reduce shadows and reflections, which increase delusions.

- Provide steady background noise such as an aquarium pump or a ticking clock in the room at night.

NEVER ARGUE! Redirect the person's attention to another place and time with a story about a friend or incident.

Wandering

One of the most troubling aspects of Alzheimer's is the person's tendency to wander away from home.

Why People with Alzheimer's Wander

There is no way to predict who will wander or when it might happen. However, some of the reasons for wandering are:

- pain

- boredom

- side effects of medication

- a noisy or stressful environment

- confusion about time

- an attempt to meet basic needs (finding the toilet)

- restlessness

- being in an unfamiliar environment

- trying to meet former obligations (to job, home, friends, family)

Wandering may also be a natural release for boredom or agitation. If this is the reason, wandering within a safe, confined space may be encouraged. When faced with episodes of wandering, try to find their cause.

The Risks of Wandering

- Of those with Alzheimer's or a related dementia, 59% will get lost, usually while doing normal activities.

- Of those not located within 24 hours of the last time seen, 46% may die, usually succumbing to hypothermia and dehydration.

- Individuals with Alzheimer's usually do not cry out for help or respond to shouts; they leave few physical clues.

- They usually travel less than one-tenth of a mile.

- They may try to travel to a former residence, work place, or city.

- They are usually found a short distance from a road or an open field; 63% are found in a creek or drainage area or caught in briars or bushes.

- Most wandering incidents occur during normal daily activities (while trying to locate a restroom, gift shop, recreation room, etc.).

How to Reduce the Chance of Wandering

You cannot always prevent wandering, but you can do many things to reduce the chances that it will happen.

- Provide opportunities for exercise, particularly when the person is waiting for a meal or an activity. Exercise might include singing, rhythmic movements, walking at an indoor mall track, or dancing.

- Reduce noise and confusion, particularly at mealtimes.

- Develop areas indoors and outdoors where the person can explore and wander independently.

- Clearly label bathrooms, living rooms, and bedrooms with large letters or pictures.

- Try a yellow strip of plastic, symbolizing caution, that is attached with Velcro® across doors to prevent wanderers from entering or leaving the room.

- Camouflage doors by painting exit doors the same color as the walls.

- Cover doors with curtains.

- Install electronic alarms or chimes on windows and doors.

- Place a large **NO** on doors.

- Place a full-length mirror on doors to the outside. Some people will turn around when they see the image, not recognizing themselves. (📖 See *Preparing the Home,* page 108.)

- Monitor medications and medication changes, especially anti-depressants or anti-anxiety drugs.

- Determine whether wandering is related to previous lifestyles. Find out how the person coped with change and stress and learn about patterns of physical exercise and lifetime habits, both at home and at work. (Did the person always react to an argument by going out and walking for an hour? Did he always jog in the afternoon?)

- Have a plan of action if wandering occurs.

- If you must move the person, slowly introduce the idea and visit the new location several times before the move occurs.

- Keep a photo on hand to give the police if an incident occurs.

- Keep unwashed clothing or wipe clean cotton balls on the person's face or arm. Put the balls in individual Ziploc bags, and store them in the freezer. (Tracking dogs can use them to pick up a scent.)

Safe Return Program

An authorized caregiver or family member can register the person in care with the **Alzheimer's Association's Safe Return Program** by completing a registration form and sending it with a $40 fee to cover the cost of the ID products. (For an additional $5 a matching caregiver bracelet is available which will alert others to look after the Alzheimer's loved one if you become disabled.) Call 1-800-733-0402.

Having the identifying information and a picture stored in a national database will increase the chances of finding someone even if that person will not wear the bracelet or necklace.

> **NOTE** Update your registration information once or twice a year, because it can be of great value to the police. The more information you provide, the better the chances of finding the individual. Call the **Safe Return Hotline** at (800) 572-1122 to report someone missing or found. If the registrant moves or goes on vacation, call (888) 572-8566 as soon as possible so Safe Return always has up-to-date information.

Encouraging Use of a Safe Return ID Bracelet

- Wrap the bracelet in a box and present it as a gift.

- Have a grandchild present the bracelet. (The person may appreciate the gesture and wear the bracelet regardless of the style.)

- If the person has a medical appointment soon after receiving the bracelet, ask the doctor to place it on the person during the appointment. It may be better received from the doctor.

- Place the bracelet on the individual's dominant hand. This will make it more difficult to undo the clasp.

- Keep the bracelet comfortable—neither too tight nor too loose.

- A bracelet that is too loose may be easy to remove. If a person is comfortable wearing a watch or other jewelry on only one wrist, place the bracelet on the same wrist.

- Find creative places for the individual to wear the bracelet. Attach it to a belt loop or purse handle, or place it on the shoe laces.

- Wear a Safe Return Caregiver's Bracelet yourself.

- If the person is not comfortable wearing a bracelet, try using a necklace.

- For someone who will not wear the bracelet or the necklace, the clothing labels, wallet card, and key chain may still be useful.

If the Person Is Missing

- Search the immediate area in and around the home first; then check familiar places and hangouts. Call out the person's name.

- Call the police.

- Tell them that the person has a memory impairment and let them know it is urgent to locate him or her quickly.

- Inform the police of the special danger areas in your neighborhood.

- Provide them with a photo.

- Describe what the person was last wearing in as much detail as possible.

- Inform the police about special medical problems or medications.

- Call **Safe Return,** (800) 572-1122, to report the missing person. Have the Registrant's ID number in front of you.

- Call your neighbors.

- Do not leave, stay by the phone, make calls brief, and stay calm.

- Call family members. They can help search and offer support.

- Call hospital emergency rooms. (Someone may have taken the person there.)

- Call transit systems to alert drivers.

- Call friends and church groups.

- Call your local chapter of the Alzheimer's Association.

When the missing person is found, call the police and the Safe Return program (1-800-572-1122) to inform them.

Checklist **Preparing for a Safe Return**

✓ *Note what the person is wearing each day.*

✓ *Have photos available to distribute to the police and other searchers.*

✓ *Have information on age, height, weight, hair and eye color, physical disabilities, and other identifying features.*

✓ *Know if the person has any medical problems or takes medication.*

✓ *Note the person's favorite places to go, "hangouts" and familiar sites.*

✓ *Know if the person is carrying, or has access to, money.*

✓ *Alert your neighbors about the person's memory loss and tendency to become confused. Ask them to call you if they see the person leaving the house.*

✓ *Know if the person is left- or right-handed. Right-handed people usually make right turns.*

✓ *Put bells on the doors to alert you when they are opened.*

✓ *Be aware of nearby hazards such as bodies of water, dense foliage, construction sites, high cliffs, steep stairways, high balconies, busy roads, fences, and gates.*

✓ *Know if the person can use a bus or a taxi.*

Information about the Safe Return program is adapted with permission from materials supplied by the Alzheimer's Association.

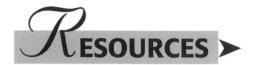

RESOURCES

Alzheimer's Association
919 North Michigan Avenue, Suite 1000
Chicago, IL 60611-1676
(312) 335-8700
(800) 272-3900
TDD (312) 335-8882
www.alz.org
Provides free literature and can refer you to your nearest local chapter that assists caregivers and family members.

Safe Return Program
P.O. Box 9307
St. Louis, MO 63117-0307
(888) 572-8566
www.alz.org
Call for more information or for Safe Return Program registration.

Alzheimer's Disease Education and Referral Center
P.O. Box 8250
Silver Spring, MD 20907
(800) 438-4380
Fax (301) 495-3334
www.alzheimers.org/adear
Sponsored by the National Institute on Aging, this organization provides information and publications on Alzheimer's disease to caregivers and the public.

American Health Assistance Foundation
15825 Shady Grove Road
Suite 140
Rockville, MD 20850
(800) 437-AHAF (2423)
www.ahaf.org
Provides a variety of written material on Alzheimer's disease.

Hospice Care

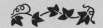

Hospice Care

Preparing for Hospice Care

Although terminal illness is a difficult thing to cope with, it also gives the person who is terminally ill and the family time to examine life, establish priorities, and renew or strengthen relationships. During this time, you can help in easing the transition by participating in choices in hospice care. A hospice team can help ensure that your loved one is as comfortable as possible during this period, and also guide the patient and family's choices for final arrangements.

When An Illness Takes a Turn for the Worse

When a serious illness becomes life threatening, a person will go through many physical, emotional and spiritual changes. While some of these changes may not be too extreme, some may be significant and decisions to terminate curative treatment, seek hospice care, or to withdraw life support may need to be made. It's best to talk over these decisions with your physicians, family and loved ones well before there is a health care crisis.

Discussing Patient's Wishes

- When possible, discuss the patient and family's wishes before an illness is in the final phase. Does the person have a health care proxy?

- Is there a living will or medical power of attorney? (See Planning End-of-Life Health Care, page 86)

- What would their choices be regarding life support?

- Would they want to stay at home or enter a facility where available?

Hospice Care

Hospice has always recognized the importance of the patient, family and other loved ones in the care plan. Caregiving for someone who is dying can be demanding and it's important for everyone involved with a terminal illness to take appropriate care of their needs.

When a cure is no longer a realistic goal, hospice services can provide expert, compassionate care and make it possible for a dying person to remain at home. The earlier hospice care begins, the more it can help and provide continuity of care. It can also help loved ones enjoy the best quality of life as a family unit.

There are more than 3,100 hospices in this country and the hospice in your community can provide information and help you answer some of the difficult decisions that accompany terminal illness and dying. Here are some questions you can ask in selecting hospice care:

- Is the agency licensed, and accredited by a nationally recognized organization?

- Are they Medicare certified?

- What are their billing policies and payment plans?

- Can they provide references, such as local hospital and care centers, institutions, and care givers?

- How do they evaluate the individual's readiness for hospice care?

- How are their caregivers supervised?

- What are their expectations of the family in sharing in caregiving?

- Are you comfortable with the program? Does it feel like the right fit?

Hospice is a concept of medical care that delivers comfort and support to people in the final stages of a terminal illness—and to their families. Care is delivered by a team of specially trained medical professionals that focus on controlling pain and managing symptoms. They provide medical, emotional, psychological and spiritual care to the patient and family, and assist the family in coping with their impending loss and their grief afterwards.

Most hospice care is delivered in the patient's home, but hospice care can also be provided in nursing homes and hospice facilities. The patient and family are the core of the hospice team and are at the center of all decision making.

Although a family member or other caregiver cares for the person on a daily basis, a hospice nurse is available 24 hours a day to provide advice and make visits. Hospice services include:

- Physician services

- Nursing services

- Medical social services

- Home health aide and homemaker services

- Spiritual, dietary and other counseling

- Physical, occupational and speech-language therapy

- Medicine for controlling pain

- Medial supplies and appliances

- Continuuous care at home during periods of crisis

- Special services for grief counseling

- Trained volunteers for companionship, errands, or respite

- Short term inpatient care.

- Bereavement services for the family(or loved ones) for up to a year after death

Although the attending physician typically refers a person to hospice, a family member, friend, or caregiver may also make the referral to hospice. The hospice nurse will contact the doctor for an order for care if that is the wish of the terminally ill person. Any terminal disease or illness qualifies.

To qualify for hospice care, these conditions must be met:

The person is certified by their doctor and the hospice medical director as terminally ill, and have a life expectancy of six months or less, if the disease runs its normal course.

Hospice care is offered for two periods of 90 days, followed by an unlimited number of 60 day periods, as long as the physician re-certifies that the patient is not getting better, and is still terminal. A patient may leave hospice care if their condition improves, and re-enter if their condition deteriorates.

How to Pay for Hospice Care

Hospice care is a benefit under Medicare Hospital Insurance (Part A) to beneficiaries with a very limited life expectancy. To receive Medicare payments, the agency or organization must be approved by Medicare to provide hospice services. Under Medicare, hospice is primarily a program of care delivered in the person's home by a Medicare-approved hospice to provide comfort and relief from pain.

Medicare pays nearly the entire cost of the services listed below. Expense to the patient is limited to cost-sharing for outpatient drugs (5%, with a maximum of $5.00 per prescription) and inpatient respite care (up to 5% of the care).

When all requirements are met, Medicare covers:

- doctor services
- nursing care
- medical appliances
- medical supplies

- drugs for symptom management and pain relief

- home health aide and homemaker services

- physical and occupational therapy

- speech/language pathology services

- medical social service

- dietary and counseling services

- psychological counseling for emotional support to patient and family

- spiritual counseling to patient and family

- respite services for the family

- volunteer assistance for companionship and respite

NOTE Hospice care as a Medicare benefit can be received for two 90 day periods followed by an unlimited number of 60 day periods. The physician must recertify the person's terminal condition. Hospice is also covered under Medicaid in 41 states, by most insurance plans and HMO's.

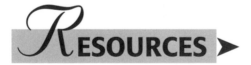

RESOURCES ▶

Hospice Foundation of America
2001 S St. NW, #300
Washington, DC 20009
800-854-3402
www.hospicefoundation.org
Provides information and referral service, resources on end of life care, search engine to end of life websites, free brochures on hospice, volunteering and bereavement.

National Hospice and Palliative Care Organization
(703) 243-5900
Hotline (800) 658-8898
www.nhpco.org
Provides information on hospice, referals to local hospices, and out-reach hospice services to families of dying people.

The National Cancer Institute
Cancer Information Service
(800) 4-CANCER (422-6237)
www.cancernet.nci.nih.gov
Provides free publications and information about cancer and cancer related resources to the patients and the public. Inquires are handled by trained information specialists. Spanish-speaking staff available.

The Cancer Page
www.mdanderson.org

American Cancer Society
www.cancer.org

Call your local **Social Security Administration, State Health Department, State Hospice Organization,** or call (800) 633-4227 **Medicare Hotline** to learn about hospice benefits.

If you don't have home access to the Internet, ask your local library to help you locate any Web site.

Funeral Arrangements and the Grieving Process

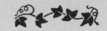

Funeral Arrangements and the Grieving Process

To ensure that the wishes of a dying person are carried out and to decrease the level of stress on the family at the time of death, it is helpful for the family to discuss all aspects of the death and all funeral arrangements while the person is still alive. Planning in advance will ensure that the person's wishes are carried out with a minimum of cost. The simpler the service the less expensive it will be, but remember that ritual is important to a bereaved family. Contact funeral homes in your area for specific details.

If your area has a nonprofit memorial association, its volunteers have likely done price comparisons of local funeral homes.

> **NOTE** People often place their funeral instructions in a safe-deposit box that may not be opened until after the funeral. It is better to keep the instructions where they can be easily located and to give a copy to the nearest relative.

Funeral Details to Be Addressed

The more details that are arranged in advance, the easier it is for you, as caregiver, to organize and administer the funeral arrangements. First, choose a company to take charge of all funeral arrangements. Then work with a staff member to decide on the details of the service and burial.

Choosing a Company to Handle Funeral Arrangements

There are three types of organizations that can be in charge of funeral arrangements:

- a traditional funeral home, which can offer a wide range of services

- an immediate disposition company, which will provide either direct burial or direct cremation

- a nonprofit memorial society association

Funeral Details That Can Be Planned in Advance

You will need to make the following decisions:

- what *type of service* is desired—public, private, traditional, religious or simple memorial

- whether viewing or visitation of the body prior to the funeral service is desired (and whether the casket should be open or closed)

- whether the service should include a display of personal photographs and momentos or a video tribute

- whether the family wants a gathering of relatives and friends to share memories

- whether there should be a procession from the church or funeral home to the cemetery

- what *type of disposition* of the body is preferred—earth burial, mausoleum entombment, cremation, or burial at sea

- what type of memorial marker is desired

- what *type of casket* is desired—steel, precious metal, or wood; sealed or unsealed; a purchased casket or one rented for the funeral (with a simpler one used for the burial or cremation)

- the clothing desired for the burial

- whether jewelry is to be buried (not recommended) or removed before burial

- what hair style, makeup, and nail polish is wanted

- who is to be notified about death: friends, family, employer, the clergy, etc.

- who will conduct the service and give the eulogy; this might be a member of the clergy, perhaps with personal statements and readings from friends, family, and members of favorite organizations or lodges

- who the casketbearers will be (avoid people with heart conditions or bad backs and make them honorary casket bearers instead)

- what guest books and prayer cards will be needed

- which relatives, friends, or business associates need to be notified by phone, letter, or printed notice

- whether the family has already arranged for ownership of a burial plot, mausoleum crypt, or cremation niche in a cemetery

- what obituary notices should be sent to local papers, hometown papers, and other publications

- what types of flowers are desired for the funeral or memorial service and where they should be sent afterwards (residence, nursing home, or church)

- whether contributions are preferred to flowers and where the contributions are to be sent

- which musical selections, special Bible passages, poems, literature, tree plantings, or other details are wanted

- who will send acknowledgment cards to people who gave flowers, food, or other special assistance

Funeral homes are not allowed to charge handling fees on caskets purchased elsewhere and can be fined $10,000 for refusing to accept them. Contact the State Mortuary and Cemetery Board for details.

Who Can Handle Cremation

- a full-service funeral home

- an immediate disposition company

- a cremation memorial society

An Immediate Disposition Company Will Provide:

- removal of the deceased from the place of death

- immediate burial or cremation

- return of the remains in a container to be placed in a cemetery (or scattered in a special place)

- help with arrangements if the family wants to scatter the ashes

- legal paperwork for the death certificate

 Most federal and state regulatory agencies do not impose rules for the spreading of human ashes.

A Funeral Home Will Provide:
All of the above, plus—

- a facility for services, embalming, and the option of viewing the body

- the expertise to help arrange any type of service

Organ and Tissue Donations

Because more than 50,000 Americans are on waiting lists for life-saving organ and tissue transplants, the person in your care may want to be a donor. In some states this can be done by getting the form from the Department of Motor Vehicles. You can also call the **Organ Donor Hotline** (800-243-6667) for a brochure or write to **Coalition on Donation**, P.O. Box 2066, Rock Island, IL 61204-2066.

- Organ and tissue donation has little effect on funeral plans.

- Anyone can be an eye donor, regardless of age or vision.

- Organs that can be donated include the kidneys, heart, pancreas, lungs, liver, and intestines. Tissue such as bone, ligaments, skin, and corneas are also needed.

- There is no age restriction.

- A donor can still have an open-casket funeral since donation does not disfigure the body.

- Organ or tissue donors are still responsible for burial or cremation costs.

- When donating the body for medical education, you still have to pay for embalming and transportation. (The remains are later cremated. They will be disposed of or returned to the family.)

- The estate of the deceased or the family is never charged for the donation.

The Newspaper Obituary

Information needed for the obituary can be gathered in advance with the help of family members. You will need to know—

- date and place of birth

- date and place of marriage

- date of spouse's death, if he or she died first

- employment, education, hobbies

- civic and public offices held

- branch of military service, rank, date of discharge

- church, union, fraternal order memberships

- names and relations of surviving family members

- time and place of services

- memorial contributions

Financial Considerations

When deciding on funeral details, state exactly what services you want and then ask for the total price of the services. Costs can differ dramatically, so make sure you call around and fully understand what you are getting for your money.

Typical Range of Funeral Costs

Often the most expensive part of the funeral is the casket, so it is wise to make a selection that is within your budget. Most caskets are purchased directly from the funeral home, but in a few parts of the country retail casket stores are available. The typical range of costs are:

- immediate burial without any ceremonies—$500–$1,000 plus the cost of the casket

- traditional funeral with viewing—$2,000–$3,500 plus the cost of the casket

- direct cremations—$450–$1,500 plus the cost of the cremation-oriented casket

Embalming is necessary if you select a funeral with viewing. However, embalming is not required if you choose direct cremation or immediate burial.

> **NOTE** These prices are meant to be illustrations. Costs can differ on a regional basis.

Advance Planning

There are many positive reasons for planning funeral and cemetery arrangements in advance. First, important decisions can be made unrushed and without overwhelming emotional stress and grief that may be present after a death. Advance planning also ensures that the wishes of the deceased will be respected and carried out. Most funeral homes offer "guaranteed" funeral plans that allow services and merchandise to be purchased at today's price.

There are several ways to pay for a funeral, including setting up a personal savings account or arranging for an insurance policy, funeral trust account, or annuity. The advantage of having an insurance policy is that if death occurs before all payments are made, the policy covers the unpaid balance. However, most insurance policies carry significant cancellation penalties if the plan is ever cancelled and will likely be more expensive for older purchasers. Trust accounts are the most liquid and in most states can be cancelled with a full refund including interest. However, if death occurs before all the payments have been made, the survivors must pay the difference. Annuities are similar to trust accounts.

Whichever plan you select, be sure that—

• it allows you to choose the services you want

• is transferable if you move

- guarantees that the original price paid, plus the interest, will provide future service at no additional charge

Other Possible Sources of Payment:

- automobile death insurance benefits

- crime victims' assistance benefits

- federal employee benefits

- funeral fund for members sponsored by fraternal organizations

- social security (a very small death benefit)

- union death fund

- veteran's allowance

NOTE In cases of poverty, seek advice from a member of the clergy, a rabbi, or a funeral director.

Information That Will Be Needed After Death

Many facts can be gathered in a person's lifetime and recorded in a simple Estate Planner. Keep this little booklet or form (available from most funeral homes, some attorneys, and stationery stores) in a safe place and let the family know where it is located.

Be sure you have telephone numbers for the following people so you can reach them easily:

- accountant

- attorney

- business associates

- clergy

- doctor

- employees

- employer

- estate executor or trustee

- family

- financial advisor

- friends

- funeral home where the funeral is pre-planned

- health representative, if other than you

- tax preparer

Financial Information to Record in the Estate Planner

In an estate planning booklet or informal list, keep clear records of the following information, complete with account numbers, addresses, telephone numbers, and the location of the documents:

- investments, their amounts, and brokers

- annuities

- bank checking and savings accounts

- life insurance with policy numbers

- Medicare and supplemental insurance

- military service and veterans' benefits

- mortgages and liabilities

- pension plans, profit-sharing, Keogh plans, and IRAs

- real estate holdings

- safe-deposit box location and key

- Social Security card and number and the date benefits began, if applicable

- workers compensation, if applicable

- list of motor vehicles owned and location of titles

Survivors' Benefits

Carefully check all life and casualty insurance and death benefits. Check on income for survivors from a credit union, trade union, fraternal organization, the military, and the Social Security Administration. Some debts and installment payments may carry insurance clauses that will cancel them. Consult with creditors if there will be a delay in payments and ask for more time.

Social Security Benefits

The widow, dependent widower, children, and dependent parents of an insured person may be eligible for monthly survivors' payments. (They usually don't start for about six weeks). However, Social Security benefits are not paid automatically. To apply, you will need the following documents:

- birth certificate of the deceased

- marriage certificate

- birth certificates of survivors (under 22 years of age if they are full-time college students; under 18 if they are not)

- proof of widow's or widower's age, if 62 or older

- proof of termination of any preceding marriage

- record of income for the preceding year

The surviving spouse or minor children may also receive a modest one-time death benefit. Ask your Social Security office for help in filling out your claims.

A personalized **Social Security report**, which outlines benefits, earnings history, and other useful information can be obtained by calling (800) 772-1213.

If you have an e-mail address, you can obtain an electronic estimate of Social Security retirement and disability benefits, as well as benefits paid to the survivors, by signing on to the Web site http://www.ssa.gov. It will not include a complete earnings history. You must know the person's name, Social Security number, date of birth, place of birth, and mother's maiden name.

The Experience of Grief

Grieving is a natural and important process that helps us avoid depression and psychological problems later in life. The stages of grief are different for all of us—and the time it takes to pass through them varies. (In general, we must experience at least one set of seasons and holidays without a loved one, but often the grieving process takes much longer than that.)

As you grieve, you may experience such intense and conflicting emotions that you feel you are going crazy. This happens to many people. However, by recognizing the common stages of grief, you can handle feelings that might otherwise be alarming. Remember, the grieving process is natural and, ultimately, will restore balance to your life.

These are some common stages in the grieving process:

- shock and numbness—usually the first stage, which can last from a few days to several months

- denial—a refusal to accept the loss

- realization and emotional release—feelings of overwhelming sadness and bouts of crying, often at unexpected times

- guilt—feelings that more could have been done

- disorganization and anxiety—confusion and an inability to concentrate, causing feelings of panic

- memory flashbacks—sudden flashbacks of both good and bad memories

- loneliness and depression—a long period of overwhelming sadness and loss of interest in things that once gave pleasure

- anger and resentment—at the doctors, the family, friends, God, and even the person who died

- recovery and acceptance—a return to a more normal life

 It is helpful to deal with grief by being around people who have gone through the same experience. Most communities have grief support groups through churches, synagogues, county mental health departments, and other nonprofit organizations.

Serious Warning Signs

Seek professional counseling if you or a family member develops a medical condition in reaction to profound feelings of loss or:

- feels strong hostility

- loses all emotional feeling

- begins using alcohol or drugs

- feels happiness instead of a sense of loss

- withdraws from all friendships

- is profoundly depressed

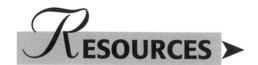

RESOURCES ▶

AARP
(800) 424-3410
www.aarp.com
E-mail: griefandloss@aarp.org
Offers a grief and loss counseling program run by volunteers who have experienced loss.

Public Reference Branch
Federal Trade Commission
Sixth Street & Pennsylvania Avenue, N.W.
Washington, D. C. 20580
For the free brochure "Facts for Consumers: Funerals A Consumer Guide", send a self-addressed, stamped envelope.

Funeral Consumers Alliance
P.O. Box 10
Hinesburg, VT 05461
(800) 765-0107
www.funerals.org
Provides information about alternatives for funeral or non-funeral dispositions; can refer you to individual Societies in the state of your choice.

National Funeral Directors Association
13625 Bishops Drive
Brookfield, WI 53005
(800) 228-6332
www.nfda.org
Provides free consumer brochures on funeral arrangements and grief counseling.

Funeral Service Consumer Assistance Program
P.O. Box 486
Elm Grove, WI 53122-0486
(800) 662-7666
www.fsef.org
Provides help to consumers and funeral directors to resolve disagreements about funeral service contracts; provides referrals and information on death, grief and funeral service.

Grief And Healing Discussion Page
www.webhealing.com
Offers a discussion group on the Internet for people dealing with grief.

The Funeral Service Center
www.funeral.com

GROWW
www.groww.org
Grief recovery on-line resource.

Last Acts
www.lastacts.org
Comprehensive website with links to resources for end-of-life care.

Write or call your local state **Mortuary and Cemetery Board** or your **State Funeral Directors Association** for information on funerals.

If you don't have home access to the Internet, ask your local library to help you locate any Web site.

Part Three: Additional Resources

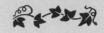

Common Abbreviations

Acute MI – heart attack

AD – Alzheimer's Disease

ADL – activities of daily living

AFO – ankle-foot orthosis

AIDS – acquired immune deficiency syndrome

ASHD – arteriosclerotic heart disease

BC – blood culture

BID – 2 times per day (approximately 8 and 8 as medication times)

BP – blood pressure

BRP – bathroom privileges

BS – blood sugar

C&S – culture and sensitivity

CA – cancer/carcinoma

CABG – coronary artery bypass graft

CBC – complete blood count

CCU – coronary care unit

CHF – congestive heart failure

COPD – chronic obstructive pulmonary disease

CPR – cardiopulmonary resuscitation

CVA – cerebral vascular accident

CVD – cerebral vascular disease

DM – diabetes mellitus

DME – durable medical equipment

DRG – diagnosis related group

ED – emergency department

EEG – electroencephalogram recording of the brain's electrical activity

EKG/ECG – electrocardiogram recording of the heart's electrical activity

FBS – fasting blood sugar, or the amount of glucose in the blood when a person has not eaten for 12 hours

FX – fracture

GTT – glucose tolerance test to determine a person's ability to metabolize glucose

HHA – a home health agency providing home health services

HIV – the human immunodeficiency virus, which causes AIDS

HS – Hour of Sleep (medication time)

I&O – record of food and liquid taken in and waste eliminated

ICU – intensive care unit for special monitoring of the acutely ill

IV – intravenous line to drip fluids and blood products into the bloodstream

LOC – loss of consciousness

NPO – nothing by mouth

NSAID – non-steroid anti-inflammatory drug.

OBS – organic brain syndrome, an injury or disorder that interferes with normal brain function

OR – operating room

OT – occupational therapy

PO – by mouth

PT – physical therapy

QID – 4 times per day (approximately 9–1–5–9 as medication times)

RBC – red blood count

ROM – range of motion

RR – respiratory rate

RT – recreational therapy

SOB – shortness of breath

TIA – Transient ischemic attack

TID – 3 times per day (approximately 9–1–6 as medication times)

TPN – total parenteral nutrition

TPR – temperature, pulse, respiration

TX – treatment

U/A – urine analysis

WBC – white blood count

Common Specialists

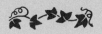

Allergist/Immunologist
Disorders of the immune system

Anesthesiologist
Pain relief during and after surgery

Audiologist
Hearing disorders

Cardiologist
Conditions of the heart, lungs, and blood vessels

Chiropodist
Minor foot ailments such as corns and bunions

Colon & Rectal Surgeon
Diseases of the intestinal tract

Dermatologist
Skin, hair, and nails

Dentist
Teeth and gums

Osteopath (D.O.)
General medicine with emphasis on the promotion of health through the hands-on manipulation of the muscles, tendons, and joints

Endocrinologist
Hormonal problems including thyroid disorders

Forensic Psychiatrist
Behavior assessment for legal purposes

Gastroenterologist
Digestive system, stomach, liver, bowels, and gallbladder

Geriatric Psychiatrist
Emotional disorders of the elderly

Geriatrician
Disorders common to the elderly

Gynecologist
Female reproductive system

Hematologist
Diseases of the blood, spleen, and lymph glands

Internist
Primary care of common illnesses, both long-term and emergency

Nephrologist
Kidney diseases and disorders

Neurologist
Brain and nervous system disorders

Oncologist
All cancers

Ophthalmologist
Care and surgery of the eyes

Optician
Fitting and making of eyeglasses and contact lenses

Optometrist
Basic eye care

Oral Maxillofacial Surgeon
Surgery involving the teeth, gums, and jaw

Orthopedist
Surgery involving joints, bones, and muscles

Orthotist
Non-medical specialist in the measurement, sizing, and preparation of foot padding pieces

Otolaryngologist
Head and neck surgeon

Pharmacist
Medications specialist; provider of physicians and patient education

Podiatrist
Foot care

Psychiatrist (MD)
Emotional, mental, or addictive disorders

Psychologist (MA or PhD)
Assessment and care of emotional or mental disorders

Pulmonologist
Diseases of lungs and airways

Rheumatologist
Diseases of joints and connective tissue (arthritis)

Urologist
Urinary system and the male reproductive system

Glossary

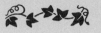

✑ A

Activities of Daily Living (ADL)–personal hygiene, bathing, dressing, grooming, toileting, feeding, and transferring

Acute–state of illness that comes on suddenly and may be of short duration

Adult day care–centers that have a supervised environment where seniors can be with others

Advance Directive–a legal document that states a person's health care preferences in writing while that person is competent and able to make such decisions

Affected–refers to the body part that is damaged or involved by the disease process

Alzheimer's Disease–a dementia that causes a serious decline of intellectual functions, including thinking ability, memory, and motor skills

Ambulatory–able to walk with little or no assistance

Amnesia–complete or partial loss of memory

Analgesics–medications used to relieve pain

Antibiotics–a group of drugs used to combat infection

Anus–the opening of the rectum

Anxiety–a state of discomfort, dread, and foreboding with physical symptoms such as rapid breathing and heart rate, tension, jitteriness, and muscle aches

Apathy–a condition in which the person shows little or no emotion

Aphasia–a disorder that makes a person unable to speak, write, gesture or understand written or spoken language (as in receptive aphasia)

Aromatherapy–use of essential oils of various plants to treat symptoms of diseases, improve sleep, and reduce stress by inducing relaxation

Artificial Life Support Systems–the use of respirators, tube feeding, intravenous (IV) feeding, and other means to replace natural and vital functions, such as breathing, eating, and drinking

Assessment–the process of analyzing a person's condition

Assisted Living–residential housing for seniors offering independence, choice of services, and assistance with Activities of Daily Living, including meals and housekeeping

Atrophy–the wasting away of muscles or brain tissue

B

Bedpan–container into which a person urinates and defecates while in bed

Blood Pressure–the pressure of the blood on the walls of the blood vessels and arteries

Body language–gestures that function as a form of communication

Body mechanics–proper use and positioning of the body to do work and avoid strain and injury

C

Calorie–the measure of the energy the body gets from various foods

Cataract–a condition (often found in the elderly) in which the lens of the eye becomes opaque

Catheter–a rubber tube for collecting urine from a person who has become incontinent

Chronic–refers to a state or condition which lasts 6 months or longer

Colostomy–a temporary or permanent surgical procedure that creates an artificial opening through the abdominal wall into a part of the large bowel through which feces can leave the body

Congregate Living–a type of independent living in which the elderly can live in their own apartments but have meals, laundry, transportation, and housekeeping services available

Conservator–a person designated with the power to take over and protect the interests of one who is incompetent

Constipation–difficulty having bowel movements

Contracture–shortening or tightening of the tissue around a joint so that the person loses the ability to move easily

D

Decubitus ulcer–pressure sore; bed sore

Defecate–to have bowel movement

Defibrillator–a device to restore or regulate a stopped or disorganized heartbeat with an electrical current

Dehydration–loss of normal body fluid, sometimes caused by vomiting and severe diarrhea

Delusions–beliefs that are firmly held despite proof that they are false

Depression–a psychiatric condition that can be moderate or severe and cause feelings of sadness and emptiness

Diuretics–drugs that help the body get rid of fluids

Draw sheet–a sheet folded widthwise to position under someone in bed to keep the linen clean and aid in transfers

Durable Power of Attorney–a legal document that authorizes another to act as a person's agent and is "durable" because it remains in effect in case the person becomes disabled or mentally incompetent

Durable Power of Attorney for Health Care Decisions–a legal document that lets a person name someone else to make health care decisions after that person has become disabled or mentally incompetent and is unable to make those decisions

Dysphagia–difficulty swallowing

E

Edema–an abnormal swelling in legs, ankles, hands, or abdomen that occurs because the body is retaining fluids

Estate planning–a process of planning for the present and future use of a person's assets

F

Foster care–a care arrangement in which a person lives in a private home with a primary caregiver and 4 or 5 other people

G

Geriatric–refers to people 65 or older

Guardian–the one who is designated as having protective care of another person or that person's property

H

Hallucination–seeing things that are not really physically there
Heimlich Maneuver–a method for clearing the airway of a choking person
Hemiplegic–person who is paralyzed on one side of the body
Hemorrhage–excessive bleeding
Hospice–a program that allows a dying person to remain at home while receiving professionally supervised care

I

Ileostomy–surgical procedure which makes an artificial opening through the abdominal wall into the ileum through which waste material is discharged
Involved–a term used to describe the side of the body most affected by a disease, operation, or medical condition
Impaction–inability to pass gas or have bowel movements
Incontinence–involuntary discharge of urine or feces
Intravenous (IV)–the delivery of fluids, medications, or nutrients into a vein

L

Laxative–a substance taken to increase bowel movements and prevent constipation

M

Mechanical lift–machine used to lift a person from one place to another
Medic-Alert®–bracelet identification system, linked to a 24-hour service that provides full information in the case of an emergency
Medicaid–a public health program through which certain medical and hospital expenses of those having low income or no income are paid from state and Federal funds; benefits vary from state to state
Medicare–a Federal health insurance program for people 65 or older and for certain disabled people under 65

N

Nutrition–a process of giving the body the key nutrients it needs for proper body function

O

Occupational therapy–therapy that focuses on the Activities of Daily Living such as personal hygiene, bathing, dressing, grooming, toileting, and feeding

Ombudsman–a person who helps residents of a retirement facility with such problems as quality of care, food, finances, medical care, residents rights, and other concerns; these services are confidential and free

Oral hygiene–the process of keeping the mouth clean

Ostomy–surgery that creates an opening through the abdominal wall through which waste products can be passed

P

Paralysis–loss or impairment of voluntary movement of a group of muscles

Paranoia–a mental disorder characterized by delusions (often the belief that one is persecuted)

Paraplegic–one who is paralyzed in (usually) the lower half of his body

Passive suicide–killing oneself through indirect action or inaction, such as no longer taking life-prolonging medications

Pathogen–disease-causing microorganism

Perineum–area between the anus and the exterior genital organs

Physical therapy–process of relearning walking, balancing and transfers

Pocketing–refers to one's getting food caught between the cheek and the gum on the paralyzed side of face

Posey–a vest-like restraint used to keep a person from getting out of bed

Positioning–placing a person in a position that allows functional activity and minimizes the danger of faulty posture which could cause pressure sores, impaired breathing, and shrinking of muscles and tendons

Power of Attorney for Health Care–providing another person with the authority to make healthcare decisions

Pressure sore–a breakdown of the skin caused by prolonged pressure in one spot; a bed sore; decubitus ulcer

Prognosis–a forecast of what is likely to happen when an individual contracts a particular disease or condition

Prone–position of the body

Prosthesis–an artificial body part, e.g., teeth, eyes, breasts, legs, arms, hands, or feet

✺ Q

Quadriplegia–paralysis of both the upper and lower parts of the body from the neck down

✺ R

Range of Motion (ROM)–the extent of possible passive (movement by another person) movement in a joint

Rehabilitation–restoration, after a disabling injury or disease, to a person's maximum physical, mental, vocational, social, and spiritual potential

Representative Payee–a person who receives Social Security benefits paid on someone else's behalf

Respite care–short-term care that allows a primary caregiver time free from his or her responsibilities

Rigidity–a condition whereby the muscles become stiff and movement becomes difficult

✺ S

Sedatives–medications used to calm a person

Shock–a state of collapse resulting from reduced blood volume and blood pressure caused by burns, severe injury, pain or an emotional blow

Sitz bath–a bath in which person submerges only hips and buttocks into water or medicated solution

Speech Therapy–the treatment of disorders of communication, including expressive language, writing and reading and communication required for Activities of Daily Living

Stroke–sudden loss of function of a part of the brain due to interference in its blood supply, usually by hemorrhage or blood clotting

Sundown Syndrome–a period of severe confusion, agitation, irritability, and occasionally violence that occurs at the end of the day in some seniors

Supine–lying on one's back

Support groups–groups of people who get together to share common experiences and help one another cope

Symptom–signs of a disease or disorder that help in diagnosis

T

Tracheotomy–surgical procedure to make an opening in a person's windpipe to aid in breathing

Tranquilizers–a group of drugs used to calm a person and control certain emotional disturbances

Transfer–movements from one position to another, e.g., from bed to chair, wheelchair to car, etc.

Transfer belt–a device placed around the waist of a disabled person and used to secure the person while helping him walk; gait belt

Transfer Board (Sliding Board)–polished wooden or plastic board used to slide a person when moving from one place to another, e.g., bed to wheelchair or commode

Trapeze–a metal bar suspended over a bed to help a person raise up or move

U

Urinal–a container used by a bedridden male for urinating

Urinalysis–a laboratory test of urine

V

Vaginal douche–a procedure to cleanse or medicate a woman's vagina by sending a stream of water into the vaginal opening

Vital signs–life signs such as blood pressure, breathing, pulse, and temperature

Void–to urinate; pass water

W

Will–legal document that states how to dispose of a person's property after death according to that person's wishes

Bibliography

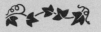

Is Home Care For You?

Anders, George and Laurie McGinley. "How Do You Tame a Wild U.S. Program," *Wall Street Journal* (March 6, 1997).

Brooks, Andree. "Pitfalls in Home-Care Insurance for the Elderly," *The New York Times* (August 15, 1996).

Coleman, Cheryl K., Carole Piles, and Marie Poggenpoel. "Influence of Caregiving on Families of Older Adults," *Journal of Gerontological Nursing* (November 1994).

France, David. "The New Compassion," *Modern Maturity* (May/June 1997).

Freudenheim, Milt. "Deductions Coming For Long-Term Care," *The New York Times* (November 17, 1996).

Keating, Sarah B. "Quality of Life Issues in Home Care," *Geriatric Nursing* (March/April 1995).

Krach, Peg and Jo Brooks. "Identifying the Responsibilities & Needs of Working Adults Who Are Primary Caregivers," *Journal of Gerontological Nursing* (October 1995).

Pear, Robert. "Medicare Denials Vary Greatly State by State," *The New York Times* (March 29, 1994).

Resident Rights When Leaving the Nursing Facility, Senior and Disabled Services Division, State of Oregon

Shellenbarger, Sue. "Families of Elders Have a Lot Riding On Budget Debates," *Wall Street Journal* (December 11, 1996).

Social Security Administration, *Medicare*

Using the Health Care Team Effectively

Anders, George. "Elderly Enjoy Better Health Than Expected," *Wall Street Journal* (March 18, 1997).

Brody, Jane E. "Alternative Medicine Has Its Place in Treatment and Prevention. But Be Careful," *The New York Times* (November 13, 1996).

————. "Pneumonia Is Still a Killer, and Self-Treatment of Flu May Bring It On," *The New York Times* (January 8, 1997).

————. "Signs of Macular Degeneration Should Prompt Quick Action," *The New York Times* (July 2, 1997).

————. "Older Women Often Get Caught in a Bottleneck With Managed Care," *The New York Times* (August 13, 1997).

Chase, Marilyn. "You Can Take Steps to Close the Leaks in Your Medical Files," *Wall Street Journal* (March 9, 1996).

————. "Not All Doctors Are Going to Shine in Giving Patient Care," *Wall Street Journal* (September 23, 1996).

————. "Consumers Need to Be Active in Debates On Medical Ethics," *Wall Street Journal* (May 17, 1997).

————. "Knowing When You Need the Expertise of a Specialist," *Wall Street Journal* (April 14, 1997).

Chavez, Erika. "Adults Still Need To Receive Flu Shots, Too," *The Oregonian* (July 2, 1997).

Cropper, Carol Marie. "The HMO Says the Doctor Is In. Is He Really?," *The New York Times* (November 10, 1996).

Freudenheim, Milt. "Not Quite What the Doctor Ordered," *The New York Times* (October 8, 1996).

Freudenheim, Milt. "Nurses Treading on Doctors' Turf," *The New York Times* (November 2, 1997).

Goldberg, Robert M. "What's Happened to the Healing Process?," *Wall Street Journal* (June 18, 1997).

Gross, Jane. "More Aids Seen in People Over 50," *The New York Times* (March 16, 1997).

Gurland, Michael S.Z. and Eugene R Anderson. "How to Make Your HMO Blink," *The New York Times* (August 17, 1997).

Herbert, Bob. "Prescription Switches," *The New York Times* (December 27, 1996).

Hilts, Philip J. "Health Maintenance Organizations Are Turning to Spiritual Healing," *The New York Times* (December 12, 1995).

Holman, Jennifer Reid. "Avoid Medicine Collisions," *Modern Maturity* (September-October 1997).

Jeffrey, Nancy Ann. "Doctors Battle Over Who treats Chronically Ill" *Wall Street Journal* (December 11,1996).

————. "Seniors Face Fresh Health-Care Choices, But a Cautious Step May Be Best Policy," *Wall Street Journal* (January 31,1997).

————. "Seniors in Medicare HMOs Should Know the Drugs That Prescription Plans Cover," *Wall Street Journal* (February 16, 1997).

————. "HMOs Seek Cure for Costly Psychosomatic Ills," *Wall Street Journal* (July 9, 1997).

Johannes, Laura. "Some HMOs Now Put Doctors on a Budget For Prescription Drugs," *Wall Street Journal* (May 22, 1997).

————. "On the Ward: Primary Nursing-A Model for Hospitals Around the Country-May Not Be Able To Survive the Push for Efficiency," *Wall Street Journal* (October 23, 1997).

Koglin, Oz Hopkins. "Blind Spot: Central Vision Is Blurred for Older Adults with Age-Related Macular Degeneration," *The Oregonian* (October 24, 1996).

Morrow, David J. "To Rate Hospitals, She Dons a Wig and Practices Her Cough," *The New York Times* (March 30, 1997).

National Institute on Aging. *Talking With Your Doctor: A Guide for Older People,* NIH Publication No. 94-3452, December 1994.

Pear, Robert. "When Are We Gonna Get to the Doctor's?," *The New York Times* (May 26, 1996).

————. "U.S. Bans Limits On H.M.O. Advice Within Medicare," *The New York Times* (December 12, 1996).

Rosenthal, Elisabeth. "When Healthier Isn't Cheaper," *The New York Times* (March 16, 1997).

Shweder, Richard A. "Ancient Cures for Open Minds," *The New York Times* (October 23, 1997).

Wade, Betsy. "Medical Care: How Shipshape?" *The New York Times* (October 6, 1996).

Whitsitt, Frank. "Who Will Change Your Diaper?," *Wall Street Journal* (May 28, 1997).

Getting In-Home Help

Jeffrey, Nancy. "New Medicare Rules Offer More Options-and Worries," *Wall Street Journal* (August 18, 1997).

Lagnado, Lucette. "A Different Age: As the Health-Care System Becomes More Efficient, the Elderly Sometimes Get Left Behind," *Wall Street Journal* (October 23, 1997).

National Association of Insurance Commissioners and the Health Care Financing Administration of the U. S. Department of Health and Human Services. *1997 Guide To Health Insurance for People with Medicare.*

Shellenbarger, Sue. "A Worker's Guide To Finding Help In Caring for an Elder," *Wall Street Journal* (May 5, 1995).

————. "Take Steps to Ensure Your Care Manager Meets Elder's Needs," *Wall Street Journal* (October 25, 1995).

Winslow, Ron. "Study Finds Crazy Quilt of Health Care," *Wall Street Journal* (January 30, 1997).

Paying for Care

Jacobs, Karen. "On Your Own: Gloria Brown Wants To Buy Health Insurance. She Just Can't Afford It," *Wall Street Journal* (October 23, 1997).

Financial Management and Tax Planning

Baden, Patricia. "Long-Term Health Care," *Better Homes and Gardens* (April 1996).

Barneby, Mary and Jennifer Kelly. "A Pension Gap for Women," *The New York Times* (August 31, 1997).

Clements, Jonathan. "Even When a Will Shows the Way, Heirs May Need Help Maneuvering," *Wall Street Journal* (May 16, 1996).

Crisp, Wendy Reid. "60 Subscriptions, and No Grand Prize," *The New York Times* (February 1, 1997).

Cropper, Carol Marie. "Vigilance Is the Price of Social Security," *The New York Times* (April 23, 1995).

————. "And One More Thing: Save This Article, Too," *The New York Times* (March 16, 1997).

Dobrzynski, Judith H. "For More and More Job Seekers, An Aging Parent Is a Big Factor," *The New York Times* (January 1, 1996).

Furchgott, Roy. "Rescuing a Relative Who Won't Accept Help," *The New York Times* (August 10, 1997).

Gapay, Les. "Crime and Punishment? Tougher Penalty May Complicate Estate Planning," *AARP Bulletin* (December 1996).

Hey, Robert P. "Retirees May Earn More Before Losing Social Security Benefits," *AARP Bulletin* (May 1996).

Johnson, Rees C. *Wills and Estate Planning*. Bellingham, Washington: Self-Counsel Press Inc., 1990.

Mundinger, Mary O'Neil. *Home Care Controversy: Too Little, Too Late, Too Costly*. Rockville, Maryland: Aspen Systems Corporation, 1983.

Pedersen-Pietersen, Laura. "Managing Parents' Cash to Pay for Their Care," *The New York Times* (June 8, 1997).

"Phone Swindlers Dangle Prizes to Cheat Elderly Out of Millions," *The New York Times* (June 29, 1997).

Romano, Mary. "Retired Americans Should Be on Guard Against Abuse From Financial Advisors," *Wall Street Journal* (March 28, 1997).

Rosen, Jan M. "Desperately Seeking Deductions? Year-End Tips," *The New York Times* (December 22, 1996).

————. "In Tax Season, 13 Ways to Smile," *The New York Times* (March 16, 1997).

Planning End-of-Life Health Care

Coker, Laura and A. Frank Johns. "Guardianship for Elders," *Journal of Gerontological Nursing* (December 1994).

Fein, Esther. "Gift for a Dying Daughter: Orders to Spare Her Pain," *The New York Times* (March 6, 1997).

Gilbert, Susan. "A Nursing Home? Or Death?," *The New York Times* (August 6, 1997).

Havill, Adrian. "With a Living Trust, You Don't Need a Mop," *The New York Times* (July 20, 1997).

Lofquist, Thelma J. "An Aging Population Problem," The *The Oregonian* (February 27, 1997).

Wade, Betsy. "Living Wills: Intent Undone," *The New York Times* (January 1, 1997).

Preparing the Home

Brody, Jane E. "A Simple Carbon Monoxide Detector Is More Than A Gift," *The New York Times* (December 13, 1995).

Giffels, David. "Universal Design Opens Homes to People With Varied Disabilities" *The Oregonian* (February 3, 1996).

Louie, Elaine. "A House Where Ingenuity, Not Neatness, Counts," *The New York Times* (February 29, 1996).

Lach, Helen W. and A. Thomas Reed, et al. "Alzheimer's Disease: Assessing Safety Problems in the Home," *Geriatric Nursing* (July/August 1995).

Tinetti, Mary E. and Dorothy I. Baker, et al. "A Multifactorial Intervention To Reduce The Risk of Falling Among Elderly People Living in The Community" *New England Journal of Medicine* (September 29, 1994).

Equipment and Supplies

Ravo, Nick. "In Some States, Lemons Can Take Different Shapes," *The New York Times* (June 8, 1997).

How to Avoid Caregiver Burnout

Bendetson, Jane. "I Am More Than Hands." *The New York Times* (April 13, 1997).

Boyd, Malcolm. "When Home Is Not a Haven," *Modern Maturity* (January/ February 1997).

————. "Sharing A Painful Secret," *Modern Maturity* (September/October, 1997).

Maxa, Rudy. "Traveling With Disabilities," *Modern Maturity* (May/June 1997).

Shellenbarger, Sue. "Meet the Bodlanders: They May Be Future In Caring for Elderly," *Wall Street Journal* (March 30, 1996).

Emergencies

Chase, Marilyn. "Heart Disease Has Different Symptoms For Female Sufferers," *Wall Street Journal* (March 4, 1997).

"Despair and Risk of Artery Disease," *The New York Times* (September 3, 1997).

National Institute on Aging. *Hyperthermia: A Hot Weather Hazard for Older People,* August 1989.

Trussell, Tait. "Stroke: The More You Know, The More Preventable the Problem," *Senior Lifestyles* (February 1997).

Activities of Daily Living

Brody, Jane E. "When the Elderly Fall, Shoes May Be to Blame," *The New York Times* (February 24, 1998).

————. "Focus Is On Diagnosis As Melanoma Rates Soar," *The New York Times* (August 6, 1997).

Chase, Marilyn. "Simple Hand Washing Gets New Scrutiny For Disease Control," *Wall Street Journal* (March 28, 1997).

Hooker, Susan. *Caring for Elderly People: Understanding and Practical Help.* London: Routledge & Kegan Paul Ltd., 1981.

Jones, Stephen R. "Infections In Frail and Vulnerable Elderly Patients," *American Journal of Medicine* (March 23, 1990).

Kolata, Gina. "Model Shows How Improved Medical Care Allowed Population Surge," *The New York Times* (January 7, 1997).

Martin, Douglas. "Wash Your Hands Immediately After Reading This Story," *The New York Times* (August 17, 1997).

White, Marguerite W., Sandra Karam, Barbara Cowell. "Skin Tears in Frail Elders: A Practical Approach to Prevention," *Geriatric Nursing* (March/April 1994).

Zucker, Elana. *Being a Homemaker/ Home Health Aide.* Bowie, Maryland: Robert J. Brady Co. 1982.

Special Challenges

Brody, Jane E. "A Self-Help Group With A Method Fights Mental Ills," *The New York Times* (January 1, 1997).

──────. "Good Habits Outweigh Genes As Key to a Healthy Old Age," *The New York Times* (February 28, 1996).

──────. "Facing Up to the Realities of Sleep Deprivation," *The New York Times* (March 31, 1998).

"Can Loved Ones Avoid A Nursing Home?" *Consumer Reports* (October 1995)

Carmichael, Suzanne. "Help Abroad In Emergencies," *The New York Times* (September 22, 1996).

Kolata, Gina. "New Era of Robust Elderly Belies the Fears of Scientists," *The New York Times* (February 27, 1996).

Marriott, Michael. "WebTV Offers Cheap Web Access, But Consumers Are Wary," *The New York Times* (February 26, 1998).

National Institute on Aging. *Age Page,* 1994.

Stock, Robert W. "When Older Women Contract the AIDS Virus," *The New York Times* (July 31, 1997).

──────. "Alcohol Lures the Old," *The New York Times* (April 18, 1996).

──────. "When It's Time to Let Others Handle the Driving," *The New York Times* (December 25, 1995).

Tabor, Mary B. W. "Path to College Degree Is Lifelong for Some," *The New York Times* (June 4, 1997).

Tripp, Julie. "Small-stock Fraud is a Big-time Problem," *The Oregonian* (March 23, 1998).

Wade, Betsy. "Airlines Adding Defibrillators," *The New York Times* (July 6, 1996).

──────. "Sizing Up Trip Insurance?" *The New York Times* (September 7, 1996).

Diet and Nutrition

Associated Press. "Calcium and Vitamin D Halve Bone Cancer Risk," *The New York Times* (September 4, 1997).

Brody, Jane E. "Good Sources of Problem Nutrients for the Elderly," *The New York Times* (May 22, 1996).

————. "Changing Nutritional Needs Put the Elderly at Risk Because of Inadequate Diets," *The New York Times* (February 8, 1990).

————. "Research Hints Vitamins D and C May Slow Down Osteoarthritis," *The New York Times* (September 4, 1996).

————. "The Antihypertension Diet You Can Live With, In Every Sense Of the Word," *The New York Times* (June 4, 1997).

National Institute of Health *Eating Hints For Cancer Patients,* NIH Publication No. 94-2079. June1994.

Kuntz, Tom. "So Let's Just Have Veggies," *The New York Times* (August 24, 1997).

Yen, Peg. "Boosting Intake When Appetite Is Poor," *Geriatric Nursing* (September/October 1994).

————. "Helping Elders Eat Less Fat," *Geriatric Nursing* (May/June 1994).

Therapies

Brody, Jane E. "A Little Warm-up For the Gardner Goes a Long Way," *The New York Times* (March 26, 1997).

Chase, Marilyn. "How Owning a Pet Can Hurt Your Health or Improve It," *Wall Street Journal* (March 31, 1997).

Doress-Worters and Diana Laskin Seigal. *Ourselves, Growing Older: Women Aging With Knowledge and Power.* New York: Touchstone, 1994.

"Elderly and Can't Sleep? Try the Scent of Lavender," *The New York Times* (September 13, 1995).

Epstein, Mark and Teresia Hazen. "Therapeutic Gardens: Plant-Centered Activities Meet Sensory, Physical and Psychological Needs," *Oregon's Journal on Aging* (Volume XI, No. 1).

Hazen, Teresia. "Horticultural Therapy: Time-Proven Art Has Become an Emerging Science," *Oregon's Journal on Aging* (Summer 1994).

Martinson, Ida M. and Ann Widmer. *Home Health Care Nursing.* Philadelphia: W.B. Saunders Company, 1989.

Miller, Robin I. "Managing Disruptive Responses to Bathing by Elderly Residents: Strategies for the Cognitively Impaired," *Journal of Gerontological Nursing* (November 1994).

"New Strain of Staph Is Resistant," *The New York Times* (June 3, 1997).

Raver, Anne. "Patients Discover the Power of Gardens," *The New York Times* (December 29, 1994).

Snyder, Mariah, Ellen C. Egan, and Kenneth R. Burns. "Efficacy of Hand Massage in Decreasing Agitation Behaviors Associated With Care Activities in Persons With Dementia," *Geriatric Nursing* (March/April 1995).

The Burton Goldberg Group. *Alternative Medicine: The Definitive Guide.* Puyallup, Washington: Future Medicine Publishing, Inc., 1996

The Road Ahead: A Stroke Recovery Guide. Englewood, Colorado: National Stroke Association, 1992.

Thomas, William. "Eden Alternative Vision," *The Eden Alternative Newsletter* (Summer 1995)

Dementia and Alzheimer's Disease

Grady, Denise. "Study Links Alzheimers to Accidents by Drivers," *The New York Times* (March 18, 1997).

Kolata, Gina. "Alzheimer Patients Present a Lesson On Human Dignity," *The New York Times* (January 1, 1997).

Mace, Nancy and Peter Rabins. *The 36 Hour Day: A Family Guide to Caring For Persons With Alzheimer's Disease, Related Illnesses and Memory Loss In Later Life:* Baltimore, Maryland: Johns Hopkins University Press, 1991.

McGinley, Laurie. "Drug Ibuprofen May Cut Risk of Alzheimer's," *Wall Street Journal* (March 10, 1997).

Patel, Smita. "Alzheimer's Disease; Sharing the Burden," *The Oregonian* (October 26, 1994).

Rantz, Marilyn J, and Ruth E. McShane. "Nursing Interventions for Chronically Confused Nursing Home Residents," *Geriatric Nursing* (January/February 1995).

"Study Finds Alzheimer's Patients Stay Home Longer If Spouses Get Aid," *The Oregonian* (December 5, 1996).

Wallace, Meredith. "The Sundown Syndrome," *Geriatric Nursing* (May/June1994).

Weisensee, Mary G., Diane K. Kjervik, and Joanne B. Anderson. "Impairment of Short-term Memory as a Criterion for Determination of Incompetency," *Geriatric Nursing* (January/February 1994).

The Dying Process

Anders, George. "Zip Code Is a Key to Course of Terminal Care," *Wall Street Journal* (October 15, 1997).

Brody, Jane E. "When a Dying Patient Seeks Suicide Aid, It May Be a Signal To Fight Depression" *The New York Times* (June 18, 1997).

Chase, Marilyn. "This Winter, Try To Avoid Taking Unneeded Antibiotics," *Wall Street Journal* (September 15, 1997).

Dvorak, John C. "No Card Necessary at Net Libraries," *The New York Times* (November 3, 1997).

Fairclough, Gordon. "Casket Stores Offer Bargains to Die For," *Wall Street Journal* (February 19, 1997).

Freierman, Shelly. "For Lifelong Learning, Click Here," *The New York Times* (August 25,1997).

Karioth, Sally Petersen. *If You Want To Know If You're Dying Ask the Cleaning Lady and Other Thoughts on Life and Happiness,* Tallahassee, Florida: K-P Publications. 1985.

Kolata, Gina. "Controversy Erupts Over Organ Removals," *The New York Times* (April 13, 1997).

Miller, Judith. "When Foundations Chime In, The Issue of Dying Comes to Life," *The New York Times* (November 22, 1997).

Nemec, Richard O. "Separating Work and Grief," *The New York Times* (August 24, 1997).

Pear, Robert. "U.S. to Go Back on Internet With Social Security Benefits," *The New York Times* (September 4, 1997).

Stolberg, Sheryl Gay. "Cries of the Dying Awaken Doctors to a New Approach," *The New York Times* (June 30, 1997).

Taylor, Nick. "An Anxious Scattering of Ashes," *The New York Times* (August 22, 1997).

Tomsho, Robert. "Funeral Parlors Become Big Business," *Wall Street Journal* (September 18, 1997).

————. "Costly Funerals Spur a Co-op Movement To Hold Down Bills," *Wall Street Journal* (November 12, 1996).

Wilkes, Paul. "Dying Well Is The Best Revenge," *The New York Times* (July 6, 1997).

Wyatt, Sarah. "Comfort and Counsel in Times of Grief," *The New York Times* (August 18, 1997).

Notes

Notes

Notes

Notes

Index

Index

Where multiple pages are listed, the main information can be found on pages in **bold** type; however, you are encouraged to see other pages also for additional useful information.

V

Vision care, 32–33—
    sight aids, 33, **126**, 133

W

Wheelchair access, 93–94, 98–99, 103
Wheelchairs—
    transfer from bed to, 280–84
    transfer to car, 285
Wills, 72

Order Form

By E-mail *mail@comfortofhome.com, or www.comfortofhome.com*

By Fax *1-503-221-7019*
Complete and fax the Order Form.

By Phone *1-800-565-1533 or 1-503-221-1315*
Have your VISA or MasterCard ready.

By Mail
Complete and mail the Order Form. Include your personal check or money order (payable to CareTrust Publications), or credit card information. Send payment to:
CareTrust Publications LLC
P.O. Box 10283
Portland, OR 97296-0283

- -

Yes! Send me **Quantity** _____ @ $23.00 each. **Subtotal** _____

Add Postage and Handling @ $5.00 for the first book and $1 for each additional book. Subtotal _____

Quantities of 4 or more, please phone for rates. **Total** _____

Please allow 2 weeks for delivery.

Payment: ☐ Check   ☐ Money Order   ☐ VISA   ☐ MasterCard

Please Print

Name on card _____

Card number _____ Expiration Date _____

Name _____ Organization _____

Address _____

_____

City _____ State _____ Zip Code _____

Daytime phone (in case of questions) _____

Signature _____ Date _____

The Comfort of Home **is a perfect gift for a friend.** Ship to (if different from above):
Name _____
Address _____

_____